Targeted Diagnosis and Treatment of Shoulder and Elbow Disease

Targeted Diagnosis and Treatment of Shoulder and Elbow Disease

Guest Editors

Teresa Paolucci
Massimiliano Mangone

MDPI

Basel • Beijing • Wuhan • Barcelona • Belgrade • Novi Sad • Cluj • Manchester

Guest Editors
Teresa Paolucci
Department of Oral Medical Sciences and Biotechnology
University of G. d'Annunzio Chieti and Pescara Chieti
Chieti
Italy

Massimiliano Mangone
Department of Anatomy, Histology, Forensic Medicine and Locomotor Sciences
Sapienza University of Rome
Rome
Italy

Editorial Office
MDPI AG
Grosspeteranlage 5
4052 Basel, Switzerland

This is a reprint of the Special Issue, published open access by the journal *Journal of Clinical Medicine* (ISSN 2077-0383), freely accessible at: https://www.mdpi.com/journal/jcm/special_issues/L5BUF7U0OF.

For citation purposes, cite each article independently as indicated on the article page online and as indicated below:

Lastname, A.A.; Lastname, B.B. Article Title. *Journal Name* **Year**, *Volume Number*, Page Range.

ISBN 978-3-7258-6622-9 (Hbk)
ISBN 978-3-7258-6623-6 (PDF)
https://doi.org/10.3390/books978-3-7258-6623-6

Contents

Journal of
Clinical Medicine

MDPI

Editorial

A Focus on Personalized Care in Light of New Diagnostic and Therapeutic Pathways of Shoulder and Elbow Disease

Teresa Paolucci [1,2,3,*], Alice Cichelli [1] and Massimiliano Mangone [4]

1 Department of Oral Medical Sciences and Biotechnology, University of the Study G. D'Annunzio of Chieti and Pescara (UDA), Physical and Rehabilitation Medicine, 66100 Chieti, Italy; alice.cichelli@unich.it
2 S. Spirito Hospital of Pescara, 65124 Pescara, Italy
3 Center for Disability, Rehabilitation, and Sports Medicine, University of G. D'Annunzio of Chieti and Pescara, Physical and Rehabilitation Medicine, 66100 Chieti, Italy
4 Department of Anatomy, Histology, Forensic Medicine and Orthopedics, Sapienza University, 00185 Rome, Italy; massimiliano.mangone@uniroma1.it
* Correspondence: teresa.paolucci@unich.it

The shoulder is a complex system of functionally interconnected and coordinated joints. Together with the elbow joint and the hand, it guides and stabilizes the reaching movement of the upper limb. The functional role of the shoulder and elbow is twofold: to provide stability to the joint complex and to allow for a wide range of motion in the shoulder girdle and, through the elbow joint, to allow for quick and precise movements. These conditions—"stability", "freedom of movement", and "speed"—are lost if any of the numerous anatomical components are damaged by trauma, inflammation, or the peripheral or central nervous system.

Rotator cuff injuries, whether traumatic or due to functional overload, arthrosis, and heterotopic ossification, are the most common pathologies of the shoulder complex, while specific tendinopathies, with or without heterotopic ossification, are syndromes that specifically affect the elbow [1–4].

From these premises, the idea of promoting a Special Issue dedicated to "Diagnosis and Treatment of Shoulder and Elbow Disease" was born, which led to interesting reflections in light of the new diagnostic, surgical, and rehabilitative treatment proposals on this topic.

Eight papers were included in this Special Issue that address the topics presented in Figure 1.

There have been some insightful reflections on the use of Artificial Intelligence (AI) [5], in particular language models such as ChatGPT and Gemini, to support medical decision making in hand surgery. This underscores the importance of assessing the strengths and limitations of different models when incorporating them into clinical practice. However, more research is needed to evaluate the use and performance of additional AI tools (Pressman S.M. et al.). In addition, advances in arthroscopic techniques for repairing isolated subscapularis tendon tears [6] have become increasingly popular in recent years. Specifically, arthroscopic repair has been shown to achieve clinical and structural outcomes equivalent to the gold standard of open repair (Bartl C. et al.). Rehabilitation after rotator cuff repair is essential for functional recovery and to reduce the risk of retear [7,8]. The review by T. Paolucci et al. found that both early and delayed rehabilitation protocols after arthroscopic rotator cuff repair can provide adequate pain relief and functional recovery. However, early rehabilitation protocols generally result in better short-term improvements in range of motion and strength. These benefits may not last, and the risk of recurrence remains a concern with early rehabilitation, especially for major injuries. Clinicians should carefully evaluate each patient's individual characteristics, injury severity, and specific therapy modalities to determine the most appropriate rehabilitation protocol following rotator cuff repair. Shoulder pain is a common musculoskeletal condition, accounting for approximately 1.3% of all primary care visits. When conservative and pharmacologic treatments fail, arthrodesis is typically considered a salvage procedure with limited functional goals. However, in "selected" patients, it can provide effective pain relief, stable motion, and satisfactory functional outcomes [9]. In the patient series by Sobhi, S. et al., shoulder arthrodesis demonstrated remarkable efficacy in pain reduction, high patient satisfaction, and acceptable functional outcomes with manageable complication rates. Considering that chronic shoulder pain can lead to significant functional disability and reduced psychosocial well-being, often exacerbated by kinesiophobia (Alito A. et al.), these findings highlight the potential benefits of this procedure in appropriately selected patients. Pathology of the long head of the biceps (LHBs) tendon is a common cause of anterior shoulder pain, including tendinitis, tenosynovitis, subluxation, dislocation, and tears [8]. In the pathogenesis of LHBs tendon instability, a shallow intertubercular groove morphology has been identified as a potential predisposing factor. Gerhardinger K. et al. suggested that the dimensions of the LHBs tendon may also influence instability, and they introduced the tendon-to-groove cross-sectional area ratio as a novel parameter to describe individual local anatomy. Heterotopic ossification (HO) after elbow trauma can result in significant motion restriction, depending on the size and location of the HO, as seen on radiographs [10]. On this specific topic, Leyder D. et al. introduced a novel classification that provides more detailed insights compared to previously established systems and aims to assist clinicians in making treatment decisions. Finally, Longo U.G. et al. proposed a minimal clinically important difference (MCID) for the 36-item Short-Form Health Survey (SF-36) questionnaire to assess patient-acceptable symptom status (PASS) during both preoperative evaluation and final follow-up after surgical shoulder repair.

We hope that you enjoy reading the articles published within this Special Issue.

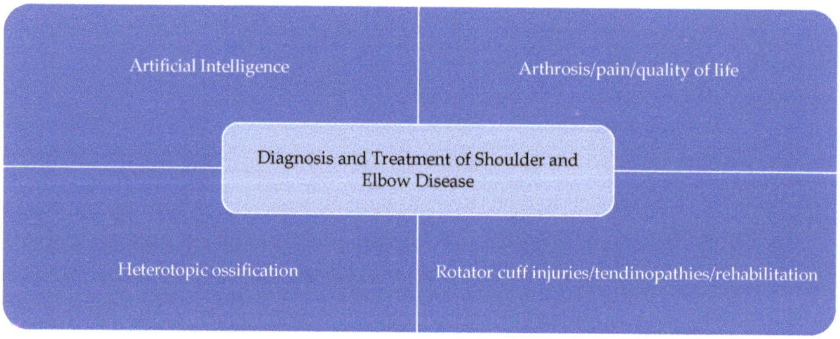

Figure 1. Topics of the included papers.

Author Contributions: Conceptualization, writing, original draft preparation, and editing: T.P., A.C. and M.M. All authors have read and agreed to the published version of this manuscript.

Conflicts of Interest: The authors declare that the collation of this Special Issue was conducted in the absence of any commercial or financial relationships that could be construed as potential conflicts of interest.

List of Contributions

1. Bartl, C.; Dolde, J.; Gebhard, F.; Eichhorn, S.; Hainzer, L.; Pauly, S. Clinical and Structural Results Following Arthroscopic and Open Repair of Isolated Subscapularis Tears. *J. Clin. Med.* **2024**, *13*, 6589. https://doi.org/10.3390/jcm13216589.
2. Sobhi, S.; Bochat, K.; Booth, G.; Mattin, A.; Moniz, S. Clinical and Surgical Outcomes of Shoulder Arthrodesis. *J. Clin. Med.* **2024**, *13*, 4701. https://doi.org/10.3390/jcm13164701.
3. Gerhardinger, K.; Klute, L.; Pfeifer, C.; Straub, J.; Hechinger, L.; Riedl, M.; Alt, V.; Kerschbaum, M.; Henssler, L. Is the Tendon-to-Groove Ratio Associated with Elevated Risk for LHB Tendon Disorders?—A New Approach of Preoperative MR-Graphic Analysis for Targeted Diagnosis of Tendinopathy of the Long Head of Biceps. *J. Clin. Med.* **2024**, *13*, 2860. https://doi.org/10.3390/jcm13102860.
4. Pressman, S.M.; Borna, S.; Gomez-Cabello, C.A.; Haider, S.A.; Forte, A.J. AI in Hand Surgery: Assessing Large Language Models in the Classification and Management of Hand Injuries. *J. Clin. Med.* **2024**, *13*, 2832. https://doi.org/10.3390/jcm13102832.
5. Leyder, D.; Döbele, S.; Konrads, C.; Histing, T.; Fischer, C.S.; Ahrend, M.-D.; Ziegler, P. Classification and Incidence of Heterotopic Ossifications in Relation to NSAID Prophylaxis after Elbow Trauma. *J. Clin. Med.* **2024**, *13*, 667. https://doi.org/10.3390/jcm13030667.
6. Longo, U.G.; De Salvatore, S.; Piergentili, I.; Lalli, A.; Bandini, B.; Denaro, V. Minimum Clinically Important Difference (MCID) and Patient Acceptable Symptomatic State (PASS) Applied to the SF-36 in Patients Who Underwent Arthroscopic Rotator Cuff Repair. *J. Clin. Med.* **2024**, *13*, 178. https://doi.org/10.3390/jcm13010178.
7. Paolucci, T.; Agostini, F.; Conti, M.; Cazzolla, S.; Mussomeli, E.; Santilli, G.; Poso, F.; Bernetti, A.; Paoloni, M.; Mangone, M. Comparison of Early versus Traditional Rehabilitation Protocol after Rotator Cuff Repair: An Umbrella-Review. *J. Clin. Med.* **2023**, *12*, 6743. https://doi.org/10.3390/jcm12216743.
8. Alito, A.; Cifalinò, M.E.; Fontana, J.M.; Verme, F.; Piterà, P.; Capodaglio, P. Tackling Kinesiophobia in Chronic Shoulder Pain: A Case Report on the Combined Effect of Pain Education and Whole-Body Cryostimulation. *J. Clin. Med.* **2024**, *13*, 2094. https://doi.org/10.3390/jcm13072094.

References

1. Mall, N.A.; Chahal, J.; Heard, W.M.; Bach, B.R., Jr.; Bush-Joseph, C.A.; Romeo, A.A.; Verma, N.N. Outcomes of arthroscopic and open surgical repair of isolated subscapularis tendon tears. *Arthroscopy* **2012**, *28*, 1306–1314. [CrossRef] [PubMed]
2. de Sire, A.; Agostini, F.; Bernetti, A.; Mangone, M.; Ruggiero, M.; Dinatale, S.; Chiappetta, A.; Paoloni, M.; Ammendolia, A.; Paolucci, T. Non-Surgical and Rehabilitative Interventions in Patients with Frozen Shoulder: Umbrella Review of Systematic Reviews. *J. Pain Res.* **2022**, *19*, 2449–2464. [CrossRef] [PubMed] [PubMed Central]
3. Li, L.; Sun, Y.; Qin, H.; Zhou, J.; Yang, X.; Li, A.; Zhang, J.; Zhang, Y. A scientometric analysis and visualization of kinesiophobia research from 2002 to 2022: A review. *Medicine* **2023**, *102*, e35872. [CrossRef] [PubMed]
4. Heuts, P.H.; Vlaeyen, J.W.; Roelofs, J.; de Bie, R.A.; Aretz, K.; van Weel, C.; van Schayck, O.C. Pain-related fear and daily functioning in patients with osteoarthritis. *Pain* **2004**, *110*, 228–235. [CrossRef] [PubMed]
5. Miller, R.; Farnebo, S.; Horwitz, M.D. Insights and trends review: Artificial intelligence in hand surgery. *J. Hand Surg. Eur. Vol.* **2023**, *48*, 396–403. [CrossRef]
6. Nazari, G.; MacDermid, J.C.; Bryant, D.; Dewan, N.; Athwal, G.S. Effects of arthroscopic vs. mini-open rotator cuff repair on function, pain & range of motion. A systematic review and meta-analysis. *PLoS ONE* **2019**, *14*, e0222953.
7. Littlewood, C.; Bateman, M.; Butler-Walley, S.; Bathers, S.; Bromley, K.; Lewis, M.; Funk, L.; Denton, J.; Moffatt, M.; Winstanley, R.; et al. Rehabilitation following rotator cuff repair: A multi-centre pilot & feasibility randomised controlled trial (RaCeR). *Clin. Rehabil.* **2021**, *35*, 829–839. [PubMed]
8. Van Deurzen, D.F.P.; Garssen, F.L.; Kerkhoffs, G.M.M.J.; Bleys, R.L.A.W.; Ten Have, I.; van den Bekerom, M.P.J. Clinical relevance of the anatomy of the long head bicipital groove, an evidence-based review. *Clin. Anat.* **2021**, *34*, 199–208. [CrossRef]

9. Del Core, M.A.; Cutler, H.S.; Schacherer, T.; Khazzam, M. Glenohumeral arthrodesis. *JSES Rev. Rep. Tech.* **2021**, *1*, 367–372. [CrossRef] [PubMed]
10. Wiggers, J.K.; Helmerhorst, G.T.; Brouwer, K.M.; Niekel, M.C.; Nunez, F.; Ring, D. Injury complexity factors predict heterotopic ossification restricting motion after elbow trauma. *Clin. Orthop. Relat. Res.* **2014**, *472*, 2162–2167. [CrossRef] [PubMed]

Journal of
Clinical Medicine

MDPI

Review

Comparison of Early versus Traditional Rehabilitation Protocol after Rotator Cuff Repair: An Umbrella-Review

Teresa Paolucci [1], Francesco Agostini [2,3], Marco Conti [2], Sara Cazzolla [2], Elena Mussomeli [2], Gabriele Santilli [4], Federica Poso [1], Andrea Bernetti [5], Marco Paoloni [2] and Massimiliano Mangone [2,*]

1 Department of Oral Medical Science and Biotechnology, G. D'Annunzio University of Chieti-Pescara, 66100 Chieti, Italy; teresa.paolucci@unich.it (T.P.); federica.poso@studenti.unich.it (F.P.)
2 Department of Anatomical and Histological Sciences, Legal Medicine and Orthopedics, Sapienza University, 00185 Rome, Italy; francesco.agostini@uniroma1.it (F.A.); ma.conti@uniroma1.it (M.C.); sara.cazzolla@uniroma1.it (S.C.); elena.mussomeli@uniroma1.it (E.M.); marco.paoloni@uniroma1.it (M.P.)
3 IRCSS San Raffaele Roma, 00163 Rome, Italy
4 Department of Surgical and Medical Sciences and Translational Medicine, Sapienza University of Rome, 00185 Rome, Italy; gabriele.santilli@uniroma1.it
5 Department of Biological and Environmental Sciences and Technologies (DiSTeBA), University of Salento, 73100 Lecce, Italy; andrea.bernetti@unisalento.it
* Correspondence: massimiliano.mangone@uniroma1.it

Abstract: Rehabilitation after rotator cuff repair is crucial for functional recovery and for minimizing the risk of retear. There are two rehabilitation protocols (early and traditional) and the debate about which is the best is open. This umbrella review aimed to compare the effect of these rehabilitation protocols in terms of reduction in pain, functional recovery, and retear risk. We selected systematic reviews and meta-analyses published between 2012 and 2022 dealing with the aim. Nineteen systematic reviews were included. No significant differences were found between early and traditional protocols in terms of pain reduction. Early rehabilitation provided better short-term results regarding Range of Motion improvement, but long-term functional outcomes were similar. Retear risk remains a significant concern for the early protocol. We found major differences between the analyzed protocols. This review suggests that both protocols are useful to recover global shoulder function, but the standard protocol has a greater safety profile for larger tears. On the other hand, the early protocol may be preferable for smaller lesions, allowing a faster recovery and having less impact on medical costs. Further research is needed to identify optimal rehabilitation strategies tailored to the individual patient's needs and characteristics.

Keywords: rotator cuff; shoulder; rehabilitation; physiotherapy; physical therapy; exercise; pain

1. Introduction

Rotator cuff tear is a common cause of shoulder pain, decreased range of motion, and weakness of the upper limb, limiting people's daily activities such as brushing hair or putting on clothes, caused by repetitive overhead lifting or shoulder injuries [1]. Mechanisms underlying rotator cuff pathology include acute accidents as well as chronic issues, often influenced by repetitive activities or micro traumas, subacromial pain syndrome, and aging; intrinsic factors such as poor vascularity and alterations in matrix composition are also involved [2–4]. We focused our research on the rehabilitation of chronic tears, often related to repetitive overhead work activities, which lead to abnormal alterations in rotator cuff tendons [5]. Rotator cuff tears are mostly found in adults and elderly people [6]: around 15–20% of 60-year-olds present this impairment as well as 26–30% of 70-year-olds, and 36–50% of 80-year-olds [7,8]. An optimal alternative to conservative treatment is the rotator cuff surgical repair [9,10], an approach that has been consolidating in recent years: more than 270,000 rotator cuff repairs are performed annually in the United States and around 9000 in the UK [11,12]. The incidence of these procedure has been rising from 1995 [11]; however, the postoperative protocol has not evolved over the last two decades, so it is essential to identify the best rehabilitation approach [13,14]. Concerning surgical techniques, different procedures can be performed: open, mini-open, and arthroscopic repair. Arthroscopy is increasingly becoming the first choice because of less postoperative pain and minor trauma due to smaller incisions through which the operation can be performed with the help of a video display for visual control [15,16]. Despite positive clinical results, reports of structural failure after surgical repair range from 10% to 48.4% [17,18]. For tears larger than 4 cm, failure occurs even more often, up to 94%, especially within the first 3 months after surgery [19,20]. The objectives of post-surgery rehabilitation are shoulder function recovery, tendon healing, and retear risk reduction. Traditionally, it is possible to identify two rehabilitation protocols: the early protocol and the delayed or traditional protocol. The early rehabilitation protocol consists of passive shoulder range of motion exercises, such as pendulum flexion, external rotation, and manual passive exercises; the patient begins these exercises the first postoperative day with a weekly high frequency. Instead, the traditional protocol is frequently based on sling immobilization and no physiotherapy: the only exception is the pendulum exercise performed for 4–6 weeks postoperatively. Another difference is in the beginning of the strengthening exercises that usually start later in the standard protocol [21–23]. A reason to prefer the delayed protocol lies in the tendon healing time, usually estimated from 4 to 16 weeks [24]. Table 1 shows a detailed comparison between the two protocols provided by Cuff and Pupello [21], who divided the recruited patients into two groups, early and delayed protocol, undergoing different rehabilitation programs.

Table 1. Example of early vs. delayed protocol.

Week	Early Protocol	Delayed Protocol
0–3	- Passive forward elevation 0°–120°, 3× weekly with a physical therapies - Passive external rotation 0°–30°, 3× weekly with a physical therapist - Pendulum exercises, 3× daily for 5 min per session - Active elbow, wrist, and hand ROM	- Pendulum exercises, 3× daily for 5 min per session - Active elbow, wrist, and hand ROM
4–6	- Passive forward elevation to tolerance, 3× weekly with physical therapist - Passive external rotation 0°–45°, 3× weekly with physical therapist - Pendulum exercises, 3× daily for 5 min per session - Active elbow, wrist, and hand ROM	- Pendulum exercises, 3× daily for 5 min per session - Active elbow, wrist, and hand ROM
6–10	- Active assisted ROM, 3× weekly with a physical therapist	- Passive forward elevation to 120°, 3× weekly - Passive external rotation to 30°, 3× weekly - At week 7, progress to passive forward elevation to tolerance and 45° external rotation - At week 7, begin active assisted ROM 3× weekly with physical therapist

Table 1. *Cont.*

Week	Early Protocol	Delayed Protocol
10–12	- Active assisted ROM 3× weekly with a physical therapist - Active ROM to tolerance	- Active assisted ROM 3× weekly with a physical therapist - Active ROM to tolerance

The evidence suggests that the early protocol may prevent postoperative stiffness, fatty infiltration, and muscle atrophy but it can compromise the tendon healing and increase cuff retears [25,26]. The traditional protocol instead can lend to correct healing but may increase the risk of shoulder stiffness [27] that is the most common complication of rotator cuff repair and a source of pain, functional limitation, and impairment [28]. Therefore, considering these premises and the debate on this topic, the aim of our umbrella review was to investigate the effectiveness of early rehabilitation protocol compared with the traditional one for the following outcome: pain, functional recovery, and risk of retear. Specifically, this paper looks for an answer to the question: "After a rotator cuff repair, is it possible to choose between an early or a traditional protocol according to the patient's characteristics? If not, could the rehabilitation protocol be based only on the demonstrated efficacy"?

2. Materials and Methods

We reported this umbrella review according to the Preferred Reporting Items for Overviews of Reviews (PRIOR) [29].

2.1. *Eligibility Criteria*

The Population, Intervention, Comparison, and Outcome (PICO) method was selected to arrange this review [30].

Population: patients with rotator cuff tear undergoing surgical repair, over 18 years old;
Intervention: early rehabilitation protocol;
Comparison: standard/delayed rehabilitation protocol;
Primary outcome: pain;
Secondary outcome: function (range of motion, strength) and risk of retear.

2.1.1. Inclusion Criteria

We included systematic reviews, with or without meta-analysis, comparing the efficacy of early rehabilitation protocol with the traditional one after rotator cuff surgical repair, published between 2012 and 2022, in English language and with available full text, reporting outcomes for at least one parameter among pain, shoulder functional and retear rates, with a clinically relevant follow-up time ranging from 3 to 24 months. The definitions of early rehabilitation and traditional rehabilitation were used as described in each study.

2.1.2. Exclusion Criteria

We excluded studies with different aims, published before 2012 and studies that considered tears caused by traumatic events.

2.1.3. Information Sources and Search Strategy

Search strategy was independently applied by three independent reviewers.

The main MeSH terms and keywords used were: rotator cuff, arthroscopy, shoulder, shoulder joint, rehabilitation, physiotherapy, and physical therapy. The search was conducted in these databases: PubMed, EMBASE, Cochrane Library, PEDro, SCOPUS, and Web of Science (WoS).

2.1.4. Selection Strategy

The data extracted and summarized by three independent reviewers were: name of the authors and year of publication, design of the primary studies included, inclusion criteria of the primary studies, intervention group and comparison with the primary study, tools used to evaluate the results for variables of interest (Pain, ROM, functional scale scores, and retear rate), and primary study references. The data collection process was performed through the reading of full texts and their relevant data were inserted in tables.

2.1.5. Methodological Quality

Three reviewers independently completed assessments of the methodological quality of the included systematic reviews via the AMSTAR-2 [31] and any disagreements were discussed until consensus was reached. AMSTAR-2 is a checklist for the evaluation of systematic reviews, randomized controlled trials and non-randomized studies focusing on health care interventions effectiveness. It consists of 16 Items with the following answer options: "Yes", "No", "Yes, in part". The AMSTAR-2 model is not intended to generate an overall score; however, a score of 1 was assigned to each item if the answer was "Yes", while the score is null if other answers were given. The quality of the systematic reviews is established on three levels: 0–5 Low, 6–10 Medium, and 11–16 High.

3. Results

A total of 19 systematic reviews were included (Figure 1), comparing Early rehabilitation Protocol (EP) versus Traditional rehabilitation Protocols (TP). Where detectable, we reported on the text the information about the size of the lesions and the surgical techniques. Table 2 shows the methodological quality of the included reviews, assessed according to the AMSTAR-2 criteria [31], while Table 3 shows the characteristics of the included reviews.

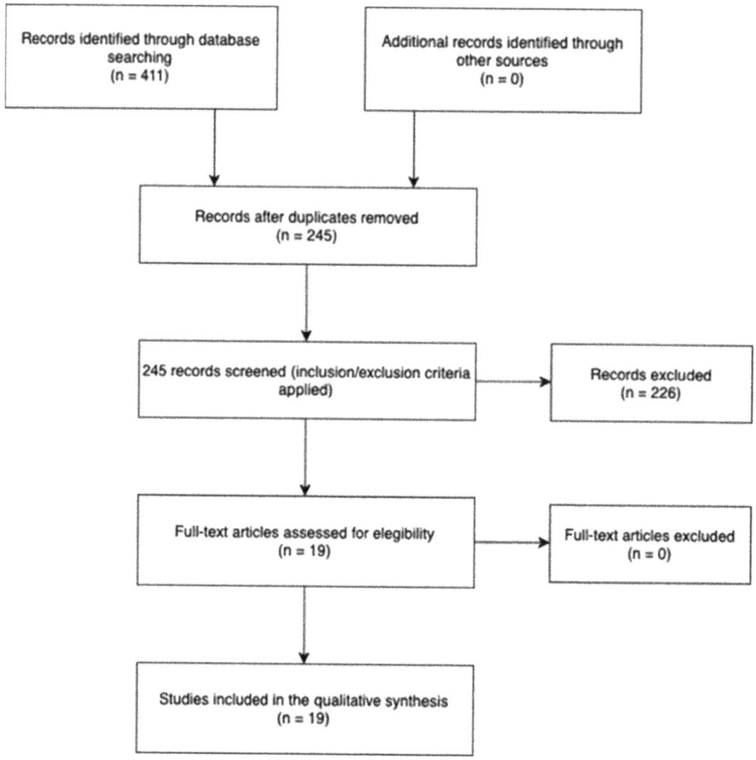

Figure 1. Flowchart.

Table 2. AMSTAR-2 criteria.

Authors	q1	q2	q3	q4	q5	q6	q7	q8	q9	q10	q11	q12	q13	q14	q15	q16
Bandara et al. [32] **(2021)**	yes	partial yes	yes	partial yes	yes	yes	no	partial yes	no	no	yes	no	no	yes	no	no
Houck et al. [33] **(2017)**	no	partial yes	yes	partial yes	yes	yes	no	partial yes	no	no	yes	no	yes	yes	no	yes
Li et al. [34] **(2017)**	yes	partial yes	yes	partial yes	yes	yes	Partial Yes	yes	yes	no	yes	yes	yes	yes	yes	yes
Littlewood et al. [35] **(2014)**	yes	partial yes	yes	partial yes	no	no	no	yes	no	yes	no-meta	no-meta	no	no	no-meta	no
Longo et al. [36] **(2021)**	yes	partial yes	yes	partial yes	yes	yes	no	yes	yes	yes	yes	yes	yes	yes	yes	yes
Longo et al. [37] **(2021)**	yes	partial yes	yes	partial yes	yes	yes	no	yes	yes	no	yes	yes	yes	yes	yes	yes
Matlak et al. [38] **(2021)**	no	partial yes	yes	partial yes	yes	yes	no	yes	no	no	no-meta	no-meta	yes	no	no-meta	yes
Mazuquin et al. [12] **(2021)**	yes	partial yes	yes	partial yes	yes	yes	yes	yes	yes	no	yes	yes	yes	yes	yes	yes
Saltzman et al. [39] **(2017)**	no	partial yes	yes	partial yes	yes	yes	no	no	no	yes	no-meta	no-meta	no	yes	no-meta	no
Silveira et al. [40] **(2021)**	yes	partial yes	yes	partial yes	yes	yes	partial yes	yes	yes	yes	yes	yes	yes	yes	yes	no
Thomson et al. [41] **(2015)**	yes	partial yes	yes	yes	yes	yes	partial yes	partial yes	no	no	no-meta	no-meta	no	no	no-meta	yes
Gallagher et al. [42] **(2015)**	yes	yes	yes	yes	no	no	no	yes	yes	no	no meta	no meta	yes	yes	no meta	yes
Chang et al. [43] **(2014)**	yes	yes	yes	yes	yes	yes	partial yes	yes	yes	no	yes	yes	yes	yes	yes	yes
Chan et al. [44] **(2014)**	yes	yes	yes	yes	yes	yes	yes	yes	partial yes	no	yes	yes	no	yes	yes	no
Shen et al. [45] **(2014)**	yes	yes	yes	yes	yes	yes	no	partial yes	yes	no	yes	yes	no	yes	yes	no
Huang et al. [46] **(2013)**	yes	partial yes	yes	yes	yes	no	no	yes	no	no	no	yes	no	yes	no	no
Riboh et al. [47] **(2014)**	yes	yes	yes	yes	yes	yes	no	yes	yes	no	no	yes	yes	yes	yes	yes
Kluczynski et al. [48] **(2014)**	yes	yes	yes	yes	no	no	no	partial yes	no	no	yes	no	no	yes	no	yes
Kluczynski et al. [49] **(2015)**	yes	yes	yes	yes	yes	yes	no	yes	no	no	no	no	no	yes	no	yes

Table 3. Characteristics of the included reviews.

	Article Type	Population	Evaluation Time	Results	Outcomes and Scales	Conclusions	Limitations
Bandara et al. [32]	Systematic review (6 RCT)	531 patients Diagnosis: All participants received rotator cuff repair Average age and DS: non specified. M = non specified F = non specified	T0 = first postoperative day T1 = 6 month after rotator cuff repair T2 = 12 month after rotator cuff repair	=ROM EP > Constant-Murley Score (no increased risk of recurrence)	Joints balance = ROM. Function = Constant-Murley Shoulder Score. Structure = Recurrence rate	(1) EP = TP—ROM. (2) EP > risk of recurrence but > functional recovery (3) EP = TP—safe and reproducible results in the short and long term.	1 Variable design of each individual study. 2 High heterogeneity revealed in pooled analyses. 3 Variability in the description of each rehabilitation protocol and timing 4 Possibility of bias in a number of the included studies
Houck et al. [33]	Systematic review (7 RCT)	5896 patients Diagnosis: All participants received rotator cuff repair Average age: 46–59 years DS: non specified M = non specified F = non specified	T0 = first postoperative day T1 = 6 month after rotator cuff repair T2 = 12 month after rotator cuff repair T3 = 24 month after rotator cuff repair	EP > ROM EP > risk of recurrence TP > Cure rate TP > ASES score EP > small injuries TP > large injuries	joints balance = ROM. Function = ASES score. Structure = Recurrence rate	(1) EP > ROM but >risk of recurrence	1 lack of reporting follow-up results, age, sex, tear size, and the rotator cuff muscles involved. 2 surgical techniques inconsistently reported in the included studies. 3 risks of bias in the ROM reported due to a lack of blinding.
Li et al. [34] **(2017)**	Systematic review (8 RCT)	671 patients Diagnosis: All participants received rotator cuff repair Average age: 58.1 ± 3.9 DS M = non specified F = non specified	T0 = first postoperative day T1 = 3 month after rotator cuff repair T2 = 6 month after rotator cuff repair T3 = 12–24 month after rotator cuff repair	EP > ROM =cure rate, ASES at T2, SST, Constant-Murley score TP > ASES at T3	joints balance = ROM. Function = Constant-Murley Shoulder Score, ASES, SST. Structure = Recurrence rate	(1) EP > ROM but <shoulder functionality (2) EP < cure rate for large injuries	1 number of trials relatively small 2 no high quality of evidence in all outcomes 3 outcome assessors were not blinded to rehabilitation protocol. 4 the standard deviation is not provided in some included studies.
Littlewood et al. [35] **(2014)**	Systematic review (12 RCT)	819 patients Diagnosis: All participants received rotator cuff repair Average age: 58.1 DS: non specified M = 430 F = 389	T0 = first postoperative day T1 = 3 month after rotator cuff repair T2 = 6 month after rotator cuff repair T3 = 12 month after rotator cuff repair	=pain, risk of recurrence and disability	Function = pain, disability Structure = Recurrence rate	(1) EP = TP	1 small mean number of included participants per trial 2 only one reviewer identified relevant studies, extracted data, and synthesized the findings.
Longo et al. [36] **(2021)**	Systematic review (16 RCT)	1424 patients Diagnosis: All participants received rotator cuff repair Average age: 56.1 ± 8.7 DS PP56.6 ± 9 DS PT M = 776 F = 648	T0 = first postoperative day T1 = 3 month after rotator cuff repair T2 = 6 month after rotator cuff repair T3 = 12 month after rotator cuff repair T4 = 24 month after rotator cuff repair	EP > ROM external rotation at T1. EP > ROM T2. =ROM at T4. =risk of recurrence and Constant-Murley score	joints balance = ROM. Function = Constant-Murley Shoulder Score. Structure = Recurrence rate	(1) = recurrence rate between the 2 groups (2) EP > external rotation at 3- and 6-months follow-up, but = at 24	1 lack of information on the RC tear characteristics 2 muscle atrophy and fatty infiltration were not specified in most of the included articles. 3 Different early protocols in terms of exercise and timing

Table 3. *Cont.*

	Article Type	Population	Evaluation Time	Results	Outcomes and Scales	Conclusions	Limitations
Longo et al. [37] **(2021)**	Systematic review (31 RCT)	5109 patients Diagnosis: All participants received rotator cuff repair Average age: 58.2 years ± 3.7 DS M = 2396. F = 2231	T0 = first postoperative day T1 = 3 month after rotator cuff repair T2 = 6 month after rotator cuff repair T3 = 12 month after rotator cuff repairT4 = 24 month after rotator cuff repair	=immobilization period =passive ROM EP active ROM > risk of recurrence TP complete active ROM > risk of recurrence =strengthening exercises	Structure = Recurrence rate	(1) = recurrence rate for immobilization, passive ROM, and force exercises. (2) EP active ROM > recurrence rate (3) TP full active ROM > recurrence rate	1 insufficient number of studies reporting the preoperative tear size. 2 no conclusions regarding clinical outcomes were made.
Matlak et al. [38] **(2021)**	Systematic review (22 RCT)	1782 patients	T0 = first postoperative day	EP > ROM;	joints balance = ROM;	(1) EP = reduced risk of stiffness, improves ROM and function faster	1 Lack of high quality studies about subscapularis rehabilitation
		Diagnosis: All participants received rotator cuff repair	T1 = 6 weeks after rotator cuff repair	EP > Function	Structure = Recurrence rate, rigidity	(2) TP = Reduced risk of recurrence.	
		Average age: 45–64.8 years	T2 = 3 month after rotator cuff repair	EP < Rigidity	Structure = strength	(3) CPM can accelerate ROM gain but does not improve long-term results.	2 Literature gaps about optimal dosage of frequency and intensity of exercise, ideal time to begin loading.
		DS: non specified	T3 = 6 month after rotator cuff repair	TP < risk of recurrence		(4) Early isometric loading may be beneficial for increasing strength and tendon shaping but requires further research	
		M = non specified		EP > strength			
		F = non specified					
Mazuquin et al. [12] **(2021)**	Systematic review (20 RCT)	1841 patients	T0 = first postoperative day	=VAS;	joints balance = ROM;	(1) EP > ROM and same tendon integrity	1 The majority of the RCTs were considered of high or unclear overall risk of bias, had small sample sizes and their definition of early and delayed rehabilitation were not consistent
		Diagnosis: All participants received rotator cuff repair	T1 = 6 weeks after rotator cuff repair	=ASES, Constant-Murley, SST, WORC;	Function = ASES, Constant-Murley Shoulder Score, SST, WORC; SANE;		2 subgroup analyses were not possible due to the lack of data reported by tear size
		Average age: 54–65.4 years	T2 = 3 month after rotator cuff repair	EP > SANE Score;	Structure = strength, tendon integrity		
		DS: non specified	T3 = 6 month after rotator cuff repair	=Strength, tendon integrity			
		M = non specified	T4 = 1 year after rotator cuff repair	EP > ROM short term			
		F = non specified	T5 = 2 years after rotator cuff repair	TP > rigidity long term			

Table 3. *Cont.*

	Article Type	Population	Evaluation Time	Results	Outcomes and Scales	Conclusions	Limitations
Saltzman et al. [39] **(2017)**	Systematic review (9 RCT)	265 – 2251 patients	T0 = first postoperative day	=tendon healing, risk of recurrence, functional outcomes, and strength	joints balance = ROM;	(1) EP > ROM	Difficulty in controlling for heterogeneity, small sample sizes and narrow study populations, lack of blinding in individual studies
		Diagnosis: All participants received rotator cuff repair	T1 = 6 month after rotator cuff repair	EP > ROM;	Function = ASES, Constant-Murley, SST, WORC;	(2) = Functional results and recurrence rate	
		Average age: 57.7–60.38 years	T2 = 12 month after rotator cuff repair	EP > risk of recurrence for large injuries	Structure = Recurrence rate and recovery rate	(3) EP > Recurrence rate for large injuries	
		DS: non specified					
		M = non specified					
		F = non specified					
Silveira et al. [40] **(2021)**	Systematic review (8 RCT)	756 patients	T0 = first postoperative day	=pain, strength, and integrity	joints balance = ROM;	(1) EP > freedom of movement of the shoulder but worse quality of life;	Different tear size and surgical techniques
		Diagnosis: All participants received rotator cuff repair	T1 = 6 weeks after rotator cuff repair	TP > WORC Index at T1,	Function = WORC Index, Constant-Murley score;	(2) Differences between groups do not appear to be clinically important	
		Average age: 50.43–57.68 years	T2 = 3 month after rotator cuff repair	=in other follow-up times	Structure = strength, tendon integrity		
		DS: non specified	T3 = 6 month after rotator cuff repair	=Constant-Murley score;			
		M = 442;	T4 = 1 year after rotator cuff repair	EP > ROM at T1, = in other follow-up times			
		F = 344.	T5 = 2 years after rotator cuff repair				
Thomson et al. [41] **(2015)**	Systematic review (11 RCT)	706 patients	T0 = first postoperative day	EP > ROM	joints balance = ROM	(1) EP = TP	1 Data extracted by only one reviewer 2 Language and publication bias
		Diagnosis: All participants received rotator cuff repair	T1 = 6 month after rotator cuff repair	TP > large injuries			
		Average age: 58.1 years	T2 = 12 month after rotator cuff repair				
		DS: non specified					
		M = non specified					
		F = non specified					

Table 3. *Cont.*

	Article Type	Population	Evaluation Time	Results	Outcomes and Scales	Conclusions	Limitations
Gallagher et al. [42] **(2015)**	Systematic review (6 RCT)	80 patients	T0 = first postoperative day	=risk of recurrence, PAIN	Function: Constant shoulder score, ASES, SST, UCLA, and DASH score	EP better ROM in short term, but =in long term	1 lack of uniform, prospective trials comparing similar rehabilitation protocols 2 All studies suffered from an intrinsic inability to properly blind individuals and several suffered from inadequate randomization or insufficient incomplete outcome reporting
		Diagnosis: All participants received rotator cuff repair	T1 = 3 month after rotator cuff repair	EP > ROM at T2, = ROM at T3			
		Average age: 54.5–63.2	T2 = 6 month after rotator cuff repair	=stiffness, =healing			
		DS: non specified	T3 = 12 month after rotator cuff repair	=ASES, SST, DASH			
		M = non specified		EP > UCLA at T1, but = at T2 and T3			
		F = non specified					
Chang et al. [43] **(2014)**	Systematic review (6 RCT)	482 patients	T0 = closest day to surgery	=external rotation range	Function = UCLA and Constant	Early ROM exercises improve postoperative stiffness but improper tendon healing in large-sized tears	1 Small numbers of included trials
		Diagnosis: All participants received rotator cuff repair	T1 = 6 month after rotator cuff repair	EP > shoulder forward flexion range at T1 and T2			2 heterogeneities among the included articles regarding the severity of the rotator cuff tears, surgical techniques, and functional outcome assessment scales
		Average age: 54.5–63.5	T2 = 12 month after rotator cuff repair	EP > recurrency	Structure = recurrence rate		3 not all the included trials reported
		DS: non specified		EP = reduce stiffness			reoperation rate
		M = 233					
		F = 249					
Chan et al. [44] **(2014)**	Systematic review (4 RCT)	370 patients	T0 = closest day to surgery	=ASES (4 RCT), CMS (2 RCT), SST, WORC	Function = ASES, Constant, SST, WORC, DASH	No statistically significant differences in functional outcomes scores, relative risks of recurrent rotator cuff tears	1 Unavailable data for several studies included in the review.

Table 3. *Cont.*

	Article Type	Population	Evaluation Time	Results	Outcomes and Scales	Conclusions	Limitations
		Diagnosis: All participants received rotator cuff repair	T1 = latest time point in all trials	=recurrence	Structure = recurrence rate		2 None of the outcomes were judged to be of high quality by the author
		Average age: 65		=ROM	Joint balance = ROM		3 Lack of blinding
		DS: non specified					
		M = 203					
		F = 167					
Shen et al. [45] (**2014**)	Systematic review (3 RCT)	265 patients	T0 = day one postoperatory	EP > Constant (1 RTC) at 12 months	Function = ASES, Constant, SST	No significant differences in tendon healing. EP > external rotation at six moths but no at 1 year	1 small number of rcTs included
		Diagnosis: All participants received rotator cuff repair	T1 = 6 months	=ASES, SST e VAS	Pain = VAS	EP Fastest ROM recovery	2 some clinical heterogeneity among trials
		Average age: 55.3–63.5	T2 = 12 months	=tendon healing			
		DS: non specified		=ROM			
Huang et al. [46] (**2013**)	Systematic review (6 RCT)	448 patients	T0 = day one postoperatory	EP > ROM	Function: DASH, Constant, ASES, SST	EP > ROM but greater risk of un-healing or re-tearing	1 few article with variable outcome measures and time points of follow-up
		Diagnosis: All participants received rotator cuff repair	T1 = 6 months	EP > function	Pain = VAS		2 data of some studies did not fit normal distributions and could not be calculated
		Average age: 55–63	T2 = 12 months	TP > healing	Structure = healing		
		DS: non specified		EP > risk of retear			3 all articles were only of fair quality
				EP > VAS at week 5 and 16, but EP = TP			
				at T1 and T2			
Riboh et al. [47] (**2014**)	Systematic review (5 RCT)	451 patients	T0 = day one postoperatory		Function = Constant, SST, ASES, UCLA	EP > shoulder forward flexion at 3/6/12 months, external rotation only at 3 months	1 methodologic limitations and moderate risk of bias of 3 of the 5 randomized studies included

Table 3. *Cont.*

	Article Type	Population	Evaluation Time	Results	Outcomes and Scales	Conclusions	Limitations
		Diagnosis: All participants received rotator cuff repair	T1 = 3 months	=recurrence	Pain = VAS	=recurrency	2 all of the studies suffered from performance bias because neither surgeons nor patients could be blinded to the treatment-group assignment.
		Average age: 54.8–63.2	T2 = 6 months	EP > ROM	Structure = healing		3 All 5 studies provide only Level II data
		DS: non specified	T3 = 12 months				
Kluczynski et al. [48] 2014	Meta Analysis (28 RCT)	1729 patients	T0 = day one postoperatory	EP > risk of retear >5 cm	Structure = recurrence rate, healing	EP greater risk of retear for >5 cm tears, TP greater risk of <3 cm tears	1 RC healing as only outcome examined
		Diagnosis: All participants received rotator cuff repair	T1 = latest time point in all trials	TP > risk of retear <3 cm			2 Most studies included in this review provided evidence levels of 2 to 4
							3 Focused only on passive ROM
		Average age: non specified					
		DS: non specified					
Kluczynski et al. [49] 2015	Meta Analysis (37 RCT)	2251 patients	T0 = day one postoperatory	EP > risk of retear	Structure = recurrence rate, healing	EP greater risk of retear for >5 cm tears ad <3 cm tears	1 RC healing as only outcome examined
		Diagnosis: All participants received rotator cuff repair	T1 = latest time point in all trials, at least 1 year				2 focused only on the active ROM component of rehabilitation
							3 unable to control for the heterogeneity of these studies
		Average age: non specified					4 small sample size of the early active ROM group
		DS: non specified					

RCT: Randomized Controlled Trial; ROM: Range Of Motion; EP: Early Protocol; TP: Traditional Protocol; ASES: American Shoulder and Elbow Society; CPM: Continuous Passive Motion; WORC Index: Western Ontario Rotator Cuff Index; SST: Simple Shoulder Test; SANE: Single Assessment Numeric Evaluation; VAS: Visual Analalogic Scale; UCLA: University of California Los Angeles; DASH: Disabilities of the Arm, Shoulder and Hand; CMS: Constant-Marley Scale.

The systematic review of Bandara et al. includes six Randomized Controlled Trial (RCT) for a total of 531 patients undergoing either early or delayed rehabilitation protocol after rotator cuff repair. A total of 42 patients with stage 2 or 3 full thickness tear underwent arthroscopic side to side surgery, 124 patients with full thickness tear < 30 mm in width underwent arthroscopic double row surgery, 130 patients with small to large tear size underwent arthroscopic single or double row surgery, 103 patients with full thickness tear underwent arthroscopic single row surgery, the data about the remaining 132 patients were not reported. The results suggest a major functional outcome in the EP, durable for the first six months after surgery, but in the long-term this superiority is not so evident. No statistical significance was found for the recurrence retear risk after EP [32]. Houck et al. collected seven RCTs, that included a population with an average age of 46–59 years, showing a better ROM in the patients submitted to the EP: this lends to a reduction in recovery time but an increased risk of recurrence [33]. The meta-analysis by Li et al. put together eight RCT including 92 patients with partial and full thickness tear, undergoing single or double row arthroscopic surgery, 68 patients with full thickness tear undergoing transosseous equivalent suture-bridge, 105 patients with full thickness tear (<3 cm) undergoing single row or double row or suture-bridge fixation, 64 patients with full thickness tear (1–5 cm) undergoing single row arthroscopy, 114 patients with full thickness tear (<3 cm) undergoing single row surgery, 40 patients with full thickness tear (1–5 cm) undergoing side-to-side repair, and 130 patients with full thickness tear (<5 cm). Different outcomes were analyzed: ROM, evaluated in terms of Forward Flexion (FF) and External Rotation (ER), proved to be totally better in the EP group at mid-term, while at long term only the FF remained superior. For small and medium tear, no differences were discovered in tendon healing, while for large tear TP obtained better results. TP showed superiority in the function outcome also [34]. Littlewood et al. analyzed 12 RCT, including 819 patients with any size of tear, repaired arthroscopically, with an average age of 58.1, reporting no significant differences between the two protocols in terms of function and retear rates [35]. Longo et al. underlined that EP obtained better results in external rotation at 3 and 6 months, while at 24 months the result was the same as TP. No differences were found in the retear rate [36]. The review by Longo et al. focused on retear rates after rotator cuff surgery, showing no statistical difference among the different period of immobilization [37]. In the systematic review by Matlak et al., only 13 studies focused on the protocols' different outcomes, showing similar long-term results achieved with both early and delayed mobilization. Those studies included 264 patients with unspecified tear size and technique, 206 patients with full thickness tear, undergoing single, double row, suture bridge or transosseous repair, 30 patients with 1–3 cm tear, undergoing single row repair, 73 patients with full thickness tear, undergoing transosseous-equivalent repair with PEEK, 64 patients with medium or large tear, undergoing arthroscopic single row repair, 100 patients with 2–4 cm tear, undergoing arthroscopic single row repair, 40 patients with unspecified tear size, undergoing sing row arthroscopic repair, 68 patients with full thickness tear, undergoing transosseous-equivalent suture-bridge technique and 199 patients with tear of any size, undergoing single or double row repair. Following the literature, EP may decrease the risk of stiffness and quickly improve the ROM, while TP should reduce the risk of retear. Furthermore, the early isometric loading in the EP can reduce pain: the authors sustained that the stimulation of scar and tendon may contribute to improve this outcome [38]. Mazuquin et al. found no differences between the two protocols concerning pain, function, and tendon healing; otherwise, they noticed a better short-term and long-term ROM, especially regarding: shoulder flexion at six weeks, three–six months and one year follow-up, abduction at six weeks follow-up, external rotation at three–six months follow-up, internal rotation at six weeks, three–six months follow-up [12]. In the work by Saltzman et al., eight studies showed a high level of evidence that EP can let the patient achieve an extended ROM up to 1 year, but it may result in greater retear rates [39]. Silveira et al. included 132 patients with mean tear size, undergoing unspecified surgical technique, 14 patients with unspecified tear size and technique, 98 patients with unspecified tear size, undergoing arthroscopic repair, 189 patients with any size of tear, undergoing mini-open repair, 206 patients with mean size tear, undergoing single or double row repair, 118 patients with mean size tear, undergoing single row arthroscopic repair, 29 patients with medium and large size, undergoing side to side repair. They found that patients who started active shoulder movement early after rotator cuff repair had greater shoulder range of motion in an initial stage, but the long-term results are comparable. However, the group differences did not appear to be clinically important, and rotator cuff integrity was similar [40]. The findings of the review by Thomson et al., which included 706 patients with an average age of 58.1 years, suggest that there may not exist a better rehabilitation protocol, so the EP and the TP are comparable [41]. Gallagher et al. analyzed 8 RCTs, including 105 patients with small to medium full thickness tear, undergoing single or double repair; 93 patients with medium to large full thickness, undergoing single row repair; 100 patients with partial or full thickness, undergoing single or double row repair; 68 patients with full thickness tear, undergoing suture bridge repair; and 114 patients with small to medium full thickness tear, undergoing double row repair, finding that the EP may provide an initial improvement in ROM and function, but the outcome at one year is similar to the one obtained with the TP. Furthermore, the EP may sustain a major risk of retear in larger tears [42]. Chang et al. stated that the EP can reduce the postoperative stiffness after arthroscopic repair but in larger tears may not guarantee a correct healing [43]. The systematic review by Chan et al. did not identify any difference in outcome after arthroscopic repair for function, ROM, and recurrency of tear [44]. Shen et al. included 68 patients with full thickness tear, undergoing transosseous equivalent suture bridge; 92 patients with partial or full thickness undergoing single or double row repair; 105 patients with small to medium full thickness tear, undergoing single or double row or suture bridge, and they could not prove that EP could represent a higher risk of tendon healing. Secondly, they found out that shoulder ROM in the EP was faster regained [45].

Huang et al. analyzed 100 patients with partial thickness tear, undergoing arthroscopic repair, 29 patients with partial thickness tear, undergoing side to side repair, 68 patients with full thickness tear undergoing arthroscopic suture bridge, 95 patients with small to medium tears undergoing single or double row or suture bridge repair, 64 patients with medium to large tear undergoing arthroscopic single row repair, and 92 patients with partial or full thickness tear undergoing single or double row repair. They found in the EP group a better achievement in ROM and shoulder function, but the early rehabilitation may increase the risk of retear and bad tendon healing. In the EP, pain outcome was better in the first weeks of treatment, but no differences were found at six or twelve months follow up [46]. The five studies included in the Riboh et al. review show that after arthroscopic repair of different tear size the EP achieves a better short-term and long-term result for ROM after small and medium tears repair while no difference in retear rate is proved among the two protocols [47]. Kluczynski et al. focused on the effect of passive ROM exercises after rotator cuff repair, finding some interesting differences regarding tendon healing linked to the tear size; with the early protocol, risk of retear is lower for tears smaller than three centimeters but it appears to be higher for tears larger than five centimeters [48]. Finally, Kluczynski et al. evaluated the effect of starting active ROM exercises in two different times of rehabilitation protocol, reporting that EP had negative effects on tendon healing when applied in patients with rotator cuff tears smaller than three centimeters and larger than five centimeters [49].

4. Discussion

Since the aim of this umbrella review was to examine the effectiveness of post-surgical rotator cuff repair rehabilitation protocol (early or traditional), we decided to divide the discussion into three main points: pain, functional recovery, and risk of retear.

4.1. Pain

Most of the included systematic reviews showed that there was no significant difference in pain relief between the early rehabilitation and traditional rehabilitation protocols [35,40,42]. However, one study reported that early mobilization might lead to moderate better pain relief in the short term [46], while long-term pain relief (about 3–4 months after surgery) was comparable between the two protocols. Since pain can often arise from postoperative shoulder stiffness, early protocol may be a helpful rehabilitation technique to prevent the stiffness deriving from shoulder immobilization. On the other hand, an early isometric loading and stimulation of tendon and scars (as realized with EP) may represent another mechanism for pain reduction.

4.2. Functional Recovery

Functional recovery, concerning range of motion, strength, and quality of life, was one of the key aspects examined in this review. The findings showed that early rehabilitation protocols provide quicker improvements in range of motion [32–34,39,40,42,43] particularly in the first 6 months after surgery. This faster recovery represents an advantage as it may lead to a rapid return to normal daily life and can also impact quality of life as the patient can return to working activities and social activities. However, some studies report that these advantages in ROM might not persist in the long term [42,43]: basically, it means that EP may provide a faster initial recovery, but the ultimate outcome would be similar between the two protocols. Regarding other functional scores, such as the Constant-Murley Shoulder Score and the American Shoulder and Elbow Surgeons (ASES) score, there is no consistent evidence to suggest that early or delayed rehabilitation protocols provide significantly better outcomes [12,35,37,39–42,44]. In terms of strength, most of the included studies suggested no significant differences between EP and TP [12,39,40]. Only the review by Matlak et al. showed improvements in external rotation strength using an EP [38]. In conclusion, it remains essential to customize the timing and progression of strengthening exercises on the patient's needs, also considering the subsequent therapy response.

4.3. Risk of Retear

Risk of retear represents a crucial disadvantage in early rehabilitation protocols, as stated in some of the analyzed systematic reviews [32–34,37–39,43]. On the contrary, other studies reported no significant differences in recurrence rates between the two rehabilitation approaches [12,36,39,44,47]. The main factor influencing the risk of retear seems to be the size of the tear: patients with 3 to 5 cm and 5 or more-centimeters tear sizes undergoing EP rehabilitation are those with a higher risk of recurrency among the total [33,42,43]. Only Kluczynski et al. found a higher risk for patients in the EP group with rupture < 3 cm when repaired with transosseous and single-row suture anchor techniques [49]. A possible explanation for the increased risk of retear in EP can be found in the early mobilization and loading of the repaired tendon, which might compromise the healing process. On the other hand, the traditional protocol allows the tendon to heal in a longer time before starting active movements, reducing the risk of retear. In some cases, based on our study, a conservative approach seems be suitable for patients with large tears and a higher risk of retear, while early rehabilitation could be better for patients with smaller tears who are seeking a quicker return to their daily activities. An important factor to consider is the recovery time: the patient may incur hospitalization-related diseases if the recovery period is extended and feel disadvantaged if he does not return to normal activities immediately. This suggests that the EP can be useful in reducing the recovery time and the derived expenses.

More comparisons based on other patient characteristics, such as age, smoking habit, gender, and occupation would be useful to define increasingly personalized and effective rehabilitation protocols. Further research is needed to establish the most effective rehabilitation strategies for different patients and injury characteristics.

This study is primarily limited by the fact that we did not report all the surgical techniques used for the repair, often missing in the articles included in the review. In particular, large, retracted tears of the cuff often exclude the double row technique which has proven to have superior biomechanical properties especially in the initial phase of healing. For this reason, in fact, this represents the major limitation of our article. Secondly, the size of the lesions was also not always reported by all the articles we included, as was the adherence to different rehabilitation protocols. This information, not reported by the authors, represents a gap that requires future studies. Thirdly, we decided to focus this work only on chronic tears because collecting the data of acute and chronic conditions together would have created too much dispersion since they have different outcomes [50,51].

5. Conclusions

This umbrella review showed that both early and delayed rehabilitation protocols after arthroscopic rotator cuff repair surgery can provide adequate pain relief and functional recovery. Early rehabilitation protocols generally lead to better short-term ROM outcomes and strength improvement, potentially. However, these advantages may not persist in the long term. The fastest recovery provided by the EP may bring a reduction in the costs of medical assistance for both patient and medical system. Risk of recurrence remains a concern for early rehabilitation, particularly for large injuries; clinicians should carefully consider the patient's individual characteristics, injury severity and specific therapy modalities when determining the most appropriate rehabilitation protocol after rotator cuff repair. Based on the information collected, the only patient-related characteristic that can be useful to guide the choice between the two protocols is the size of the lesion. Future studies are needed to better quantify the possible differences and characteristics that can influence the choice of one protocol over another.

Author Contributions: Conceptualization, T.P. and M.M.; methodology, F.A.; software, M.C.; validation, S.C., E.M. and F.P.; formal analysis, M.C.; investigation, G.S.; resources, A.B.; data curation, M.P.; writing—original draft preparation, S.C.; writing—review and editing, F.A.; visualization, M.M.; supervision, T.P.; project administration, M.P.; funding acquisition, none. All authors have read and agreed to the published version of the manuscript.

Funding: This research received no external funding.

Institutional Review Board Statement: Not applicable.

Informed Consent Statement: Not applicable.

Data Availability Statement: In this study no data were reported.

Conflicts of Interest: The authors declare no conflict of interest.

References

1. Littlewood, C.; May, S.; Walters, S. Epidemiology of Rotator Cuff Tendinopathy: A Systematic Review. *Shoulder Elb.* **2013**, *5*, 256–265. [CrossRef]
2. Consigliere, P.; Haddo, O.; Levy, O.; Sforza, G. Subacromial impingement syndrome: Management challenges. *Orthop. Res. Rev.* **2018**, *10*, 83–91. [CrossRef] [PubMed]
3. Keener, J.D.; Patterson, B.M.; Orvets, N.; Chamberlain, A.M. Degenerative rotator cuff tears: Refining surgical indications based on natural history data. *J. Am. Acad. Orthop. Surg.* **2019**, *27*, 156–165. [CrossRef]
4. Yazdani, A.N.; Rai, V.; Agrawal, D.K. Rotator Cuff Health, Pathology, and Repair in the Perspective of Hyperlipidemia. *J. Orthop. Sport. Med.* **2022**, *4*, 263–275. [CrossRef] [PubMed]
5. Razmjou, H.; Lincoln, S.; Axelrod, T.; Holtby, R. Factors Contributing to Failure of Rotator Cuff Surgery in Persons with Work-Related Injuries. *Physiother. Can.* **2008**, *60*, 125. [CrossRef]
6. Oh, J.H.; Park, M.S.; Rhee, S.M. Treatment Strategy for Irreparable Rotator Cuff Tears. *Clin. Orthop. Surg.* **2018**, *10*, 119–134. [CrossRef]
7. Tempelhof, S.; Rupp, S.; Seil, R. Age-related prevalence of rotator cuff tears in asymptomatic shoulders. *J. Shoulder Elb. Surg.* **1999**, *8*, 296–299. [CrossRef]
8. Minagawa, H.; Yamamoto, N.; Abe, H.; Fukuda, M.; Seki, N.; Kikuchi, K.; Kijima, H.; Itoi, E. Prevalence of symptomatic and asymptomatic rotator cuff tears in the general population: From mass-screening in one village. *J. Orthop.* **2013**, *10*, 8–12. [CrossRef]

9. Littlewood, C.; Bateman, M.; Butler-Walley, S.; Bathers, S.; Bromley, K.; Lewis, M.; Funk, L.; Denton, J.; Moffatt, M.; Winstanley, R.; et al. Rehabilitation following rotator cuff repair: A multi-centre pilot & feasibility randomised controlled trial (RaCeR). *Clin. Rehabil.* **2021**, *35*, 829–839. [CrossRef]
10. Gartsman, G.M. Arthroscopic management of rotator cuff disease. *J. Am. Acad. Orthop. Surg.* **1998**, *6*, 259–266. [CrossRef]
11. Ensor, K.L.; Kwon, Y.W.; Dibeneditto, M.R.; Zuckerman, J.D.; Rokito, A.S. The rising incidence of rotator cuff repairs. *J. Shoulder Elb. Surg.* **2013**, *22*, 1628–1632. [CrossRef]
12. Mazuquin, B.; Moffatt, M.; Gill, P.; Selfe, J.; Rees, J.; Drew, S.; Littlewood, C. Effectiveness of early versus delayed rehabilitation following rotator cuff repair: Systematic review and meta-analyses. *PLoS ONE* **2021**, *16*, e0252137. [CrossRef]
13. Jain, N.B.; Higgins, L.D.; Losina, E.; Collins, J.; Blazar, P.E.; Katz, J.N. Epidemiology of musculoskeletal upper extremity ambulatory surgery in the United States. *BMC Musculoskelet. Disord.* **2014**, *15*, 4. [CrossRef]
14. Littlewood, C.; Mazuquin, B.; Moffatt, M.; Bateman, M. Rehabilitation following rotator cuff repair: A survey of current practice. *Musculoskelet. Care* **2021**, *19*, 165–171. [CrossRef]
15. Cho, C.-H.; Song, K.-S.; Jung, G.H.; Lee, Y.K.; Shin, H.K. Early postoperative outcomes between arthroscopic and mini-open repair for rotator cuff tears. *Orthopedics* **2012**, *35*, 1347–1352. [CrossRef]
16. Nazari, G.; MacDermid, J.C.; Bryant, D.; Dewan, N.; Athwal, G.S. Effects of arthroscopic vs. mini-open rotator cuff repair on function, pain & range of motion. A systematic review and meta-analysis. *PLoS ONE* **2019**, *14*, e0222953. [CrossRef]
17. Cole, B.J.; McCarty, L.P.; Kang, R.W.; Alford, W.; Lewis, P.B.; Hayden, J.K. Arthroscopic rotator cuff repair: Prospective functional outcome and repair integrity at minimum 2-year follow-up. *J. Shoulder Elb. Surg.* **2007**, *16*, 579–585. [CrossRef]
18. DeFranco, M.J.; Bershadsky, B.; Ciccone, J.; Yum, J.K.; Iannotti, J.P. Functional outcome of arthroscopic rotator cuff repairs: A correlation of anatomic and clinical results. *J. Shoulder Elb. Surg.* **2007**, *16*, 759–765. [CrossRef]
19. Iannotti, J.P.; Deutsch, A.; Green, A.; Rudicel, S.; Christensen, J.; Marraffino, S.; Rodeo, S. Time to failure after rotator cuff repair: A prospective imaging study. *J. Bone Jt. Surg. Am.* **2013**, *95*, 965–971. [CrossRef]
20. Zhao, J.; Luo, M.; Pan, J.; Liang, G.; Feng, W.; Zeng, L.; Yang, W.; Liu, J. Risk factors affecting rotator cuff retear after arthroscopic repair: A meta-analysis and systematic review. *J. Shoulder Elb. Surg.* **2021**, *30*, 2660–2670. [CrossRef]
21. Cuff, D.J.; Pupello, D.R. Prospective randomized study of arthroscopic rotator cuff repair using an early versus delayed postoperative physical therapy protocol. *J. Shoulder Elb. Surg.* **2012**, *21*, 1450–1455. [CrossRef]
22. Düzgün, I.; Baltacı, G.; Atay, O.A. Comparison of slow and accelerated rehabilitation protocol after arthroscopic rotator cuff repair: Pain and functional activity. *Acta Orthop. Traumatol. Turc.* **2011**, *45*, 23–33. [CrossRef]
23. Arndt, J.; Clavert, P.; Mielcarek, P.; Bouchaib, J.; Meyer, N.; Kempf, J.F. French Society for Shoulder & Elbow (SOFEC). Immediate passive motion versus immobilization after endoscopic supraspinatus tendon repair: A prospective randomized study. *Orthop. Traumatol. Surg. Res.* **2012**, *98*, S131–S138. [CrossRef]
24. Peltzm, C.D.; Sarver, J.J.; Dourte, L.M.; Würgler-Hauri, C.C.; Williams, G.R.; Soslowsky, L.J. Exercise following a short immobilization period is detrimental to tendon properties and joint mechanics in a rat rotator cuff injury model. *J. Orthop. Res.* **2010**, *28*, 841–845. [CrossRef]
25. Huberty, D.P.; Schoolfield, J.D.; Brady, P.C.; Vadala, A.P.; Arrigoni, P.; Burkhart, S.S. Incidence and treatment of postoperative stiffness following arthroscopic rotator cuff repair. *Arthroscopy* **2009**, *25*, 880–890. [CrossRef]
26. Papalia, R.; Franceschi, F.; Vasta, S.; Gallo, A.; Maffulli, N.; Denaro, V. Shoulder stiffness and rotator cuff repair. *Br. Med. Bull.* **2012**, *104*, 163–174. [CrossRef]
27. Chen, L.; Peng, K.; Zhang, D.; Peng, J.; Xing, F.; Xiang, Z. Rehabilitation protocol after arthroscopic rotator cuff repair: Early versus delayed motion. *Int. J. Clin. Exp. Med.* **2015**, *8*, 8329–8338.
28. Namdari, S.; Green, A. Range of motion limitation after rotator cuff repair. *J. Shoulder Elb. Surg.* **2010**, *19*, 290–296. [CrossRef]
29. Pollock, M.; Fernandes, R.M.; Pieper, D.; Tricco, A.C.; Gates, M.; Gates, A.; Hartling, L. Preferred Reporting Items for Overviews of Reviews (PRIOR): A protocol for development of a reporting guideline for overviews of reviews of healthcare interventions. *Syst. Rev.* **2019**, *8*, 335. [CrossRef]
30. Methley, A.M.; Campbell, S.; Chew-Graham, C.; McNally, R.; Cheraghi-Sohi, S. PICO, PICOS and SPIDER: A comparison study of specificity and sensitivity in three search tools for qualitative systematic reviews. *BMC Health Serv. Res.* **2014**, *14*, 579. [CrossRef]
31. Shea, B.J.; Reeves, B.C.; Wells, G.; Thuku, M.; Hamel, C.; Moran, J.; Moher, D.; Tugwell, P.; Welch, V.; Kristjansson, E.; et al. AMSTAR 2: A critical appraisal tool for systematic reviews that include randomised or non-randomised studies of healthcare interventions, or both. *BMJ* **2017**, *358*, 4008. [CrossRef]
32. Bandara, U.; An, V.V.G.; Imani, S.; Nandapalan, H.; Sivakumar, B.S. Rehabilitation protocols following rotator cuff repair: A meta-analysis of current evidence. *ANZ J. Surg.* **2021**, *91*, 2773–2779. [CrossRef]
33. Houck, D.A.; Kraeutler, M.J.; Schuette, H.B.; McCarty, E.C.; Bravman, J.T. Early Versus Delayed Motion after Rotator Cuff Repair: A Systematic Review of Overlapping Meta-analyses. *Am. J. Sport. Med.* **2017**, *45*, 2911–2915. [CrossRef]
34. Li, S.; Sun, H.; Luo, X.; Wang, K.; Wu, G.; Zhou, J.; Wang, P.; Sun, X. The clinical effect of rehabilitation following arthroscopic rotator cuff repair: A meta-analysis of early versus delayed passive motion. *Medicine* **2018**, *97*, e9625. [CrossRef] [PubMed]
35. Littlewood, C.; Bateman, M.; Clark, D.; Selfe, J.; Watkinson, D.; Walton, M.; Funk, L. Rehabilitation following rotator cuff repair: A systematic review. *Shoulder Elb.* **2015**, *7*, 115–124. [CrossRef]

36. Longo, U.G.; Risi Ambrogioni, L.; Berton, A.; Candela, V.; Migliorini, F.; Carnevale, A.; Schena, E.; Nazarian, A.; DeAngelis, J.; Denaro, V. Conservative versus accelerated rehabilitation after rotator cuff repair: A systematic review and meta-analysis. *BMC Musculoskelet. Disord.* **2021**, *22*, 637. [CrossRef] [PubMed]
37. Longo, U.G.; Carnevale, A.; Piergentili, I.; Berton, A.; Candela, V.; Schena, E.; Denaro, V. Retear rates after rotator cuff surgery: A systematic review and meta-analysis. *BMC Musculoskelet. Disord.* **2021**, *22*, 749. [CrossRef] [PubMed]
38. Matlak, S.; Andrews, A.; Looney, A.; Tepper, K.B. Postoperative Rehabilitation of Rotator Cuff Repair: A Systematic Review. *Sports Med. Arthrosc. Rev.* **2021**, *29*, 119–129. [CrossRef]
39. Saltzman, B.M.; Zuke, W.A.; Go, B.; Mascarenhas, R.; Verma, N.N.; Cole, B.J.; Romeo, A.A.; Forsythe, B. Does early motion lead to a higher failure rate or better outcomes after arthroscopic rotator cuff repair? A systematic review of overlapping meta-analyses. *J. Shoulder Elb. Surg.* **2017**, *26*, 1681–1691. [CrossRef]
40. Silveira, A.; Luk, J.; Tan, M.; Kang, S.H.; Sheps, D.M.; Bouliane, M.; Beaupre, L. Move It or Lose It? The Effect of Early Active Movement on Clinical Outcomes Following Rotator Cuff Repair: A Systematic Review with Meta-analysis. *J. Orthop. Sport. Phys. Ther.* **2021**, *51*, 331–344. [CrossRef]
41. Thomson, S.; Jukes, C.; Lewis, J.S. Rehabilitation following surgical repair of the rotator cuff: A systematic review. *Physiotherapy* **2016**, *102*, 20–28. [CrossRef]
42. Gallagher, B.P.; Bishop, M.E.; Tjoumakaris, F.P.; Freedman, K.B. Early versus delayed rehabilitation following arthroscopic rotator cuff repair: A systematic review. *Phys. Sport.* **2015**, *43*, 178–187. [CrossRef]
43. Chang, K.V.; Hung, C.Y.; Han, D.S.; Chen, W.S.; Wang, T.G.; Chien, K.L. Early versus delayed passive range of motion exercise for arthroscopic rotator cuff repair: A meta-analysis of randomized controlled trials. *Am. J. Sport. Med.* **2015**, *43*, 1265–1273. [CrossRef]
44. Chan, K.; MacDermid, J.C.; Hoppe, D.J.; Ayeni, O.R.; Bhandari, M.; Foote, C.J.; Athwal, G.S. Delayed versus early motion after arthroscopic rotator cuff repair: A meta-analysis. *J. Shoulder Elb. Surg.* **2014**, *23*, 1631–1639. [CrossRef] [PubMed]
45. Shen, C.; Tang, Z.H.; Hu, J.Z.; Zou, G.Y.; Xiao, R.C.; Yan, D.X. Does immobilization after arthroscopic rotator cuff repair increase tendon healing? A systematic review and meta-analysis. *Arch. Orthop. Trauma Surg.* **2014**, *134*, 1279–1285. [CrossRef]
46. Huang, T.S.; Wang, S.F.; Lin, J.-J. Comparison of Aggressive and Traditional Postoperative Rehabilitation Protocol after Rotator Cuff Repair: A Meta-analysis. *J. Nov. Physiother.* **2013**, *3*, 170. [CrossRef]
47. Riboh, J.C.; Garrigues, G.E. Early passive motion versus immobilization after arthroscopic rotator cuff repair. *Arthrosc.-J. Arthrosc. Relat. Surg.* **2014**, *30*, 997–1005. [CrossRef]
48. Kluczynski, M.A.; Nayyar, S.; Marzo, J.M.; Bisson, L.J. Early Versus Delayed Passive Range of Motion after Rotator Cuff Repair: A Systematic Review and Meta-analysis. *Am. J. Sport. Med.* **2015**, *43*, 2057–2063. [CrossRef] [PubMed]
49. Kluczynski, M.A.; Isenburg, M.M.; Marzo, J.M.; Bisson, L.J. Does Early versus Delayed Active Range of Motion Affect Rotator Cuff Healing after Surgical Repair? *Am. J. Sport. Med.* **2016**, *44*, 785–791. [CrossRef] [PubMed]
50. Brian, M.G.; Jonathan, D.H.; Stephanie, A.B.; Albert, L.; Bryson, P.L. Comparison of Functional Outcomes after Arthroscopic Rotator Cuff Repair between Patients with Traumatic and Atraumatic Tears. *Orthop. J. Sport. Med.* **2022**, *10*, 23259671221126551. [CrossRef]
51. Paul, S.; Yadav, A.K.; Goyal, T. Comparison of tear characteristics, outcome parameters and healing in traumatic and non-traumatic rotator cuff tear: A prospective cohort study. *Musculoskelet. Surg.* **2022**, *106*, 433–440. [CrossRef] [PubMed]

Journal of
Clinical Medicine

MDPI

Article

Minimum Clinically Important Difference (MCID) and Patient Acceptable Symptomatic State (PASS) Applied to the SF-36 in Patients Who Underwent Arthroscopic Rotator Cuff Repair

Umile Giuseppe Longo [1,2,*], Sergio De Salvatore [1,3], Ilaria Piergentili [4], Alberto Lalli [1,2], Benedetta Bandini [1,2] and Vincenzo Denaro [1,2]

1 Fondazione Policlinico Universitario Campus Bio-Medico, Via Alvaro del Portillo, 200, 00128 Rome, Italy; s.desalvatore@unicampus.it (S.D.S.); albertolalli30@gmail.com (A.L.); benedettabandini.000@gmail.com (B.B.); denaro.cbm@gmail.com (V.D.)
2 Research Unit of Orthopaedic and Trauma Surgery, Department of Medicine and Surgery, Università Campus Bio-Medico di Roma, Via Alvaro del Portillo, 21, 00128 Rome, Italy
3 Research Unit of Ospedale Pediatrico Bambin Gesù, Department of Medicine and Surgery, Via della Torre di Palidoro, 00050 Fiumicino, Italy
4 CNR-IASI, Laboratorio di Biomatematica, Consiglio Nazionale delle Ricerche, Istituto di Analisi dei Sistemi ed Informatica, 00185 Rome, Italy; ilaria.piergentili94@gmail.com
* Correspondence: g.longo@unicampus.it; Tel.: +39-06-225411613

Abstract: The 36-Item Short-Form Health Survey questionnaire (SF-36) is a reliable tool to assess the health-related quality of life of patients. If a mean difference between pre-operative evaluation and final follow-up is found to be statistically significant, then the change in score is not random. However, a statistically significant mean change may not correspond to a clinical amelioration for the patient or mean that the patient's state of health is to be considered acceptable. For this reason, interest in the concepts of minimal clinically important difference (MCID) and patient acceptable symptomatic state (PASS) has grown within recent years. The goal of the present work of research was to determine the MCID and PASS values for the SF-36 in patients who received rotator cuff repair (RCR). Forty-six patients (18 women and 28 men, mean age 58.5 ± 12.9) previously diagnosed with rotator cuff disease were enrolled. All of these patients underwent RCR. They were evaluated pre-operatively and six months after the surgical intervention as a final follow-up. The SF-36 questionnaire was assessed at each evaluation. The MCID cut-offs of the total, physical, and mental dimensions of the SF-36 for patients who underwent RCR were 23.1, 32.5, and 18.1, respectively. A 23.1 improvement in the SF-36 score at six months following RCR can be correlated with patients having reached a clinically significant improvement in health status. If 81.9 or more is attained in the SF-36 score after surgical repair, the symptom state can be judged as satisfactory by the majority of patients.

Keywords: shoulder joint; rotator cuff repair; minimal clinically important difference; patient-reported outcome measures; patient acceptable symptomatic state

1. Introduction

To assess rotator cuff repair (RCR), the most commonly applied clinical scores are the Disabilities of the Arm, Shoulder, and Hand Questionnaire, Shoulder Pain and Disability Index, American Shoulder and Elbow surgeons (ASES), Constant Murley Score, Simple Shoulder Test (SST), Oxford Shoulder Score, Shoulder Disability Questionnaire, and Western Ontario Shoulder Instability Index [1].

To determine the effectiveness of a given surgical procedure, the mean difference of an outcome score from baseline to postoperative follow-up is usually assessed. If the mean difference is statistically significant between the two time points, then the change in score is not random. However, a statistically significant mean variation may not correspond to a clinical improvement for the patient or mean that the patient's state of health is to be considered acceptable. For this reason, interest in the concepts of Minimal Clinically Important Difference (MCID) and Patient Acceptable Symptomatic State (PASS) has increased over the last few years. The MCID is defined as the lowest amount of variation in an outcome measurement that enables a patient to self-assess their own level of improvement following therapy [2]. The PASS refers to the value that defines the patient's satisfaction with a symptom state when the pain and function are considered together [3]. These tools can be exploited to evaluate if the outcomes considered in a research work or clinical environment for a surgical procedure can be judged as clinically meaningful.

The 36-Item Short-Form Health Survey questionnaire (SF-36) is a reliable tool to assess health-related quality of life, and it is broadly exploited in orthopedic-related research [4]. The SF-36 questionnaire is a 36-item health survey that considers eight different dimensions of health. These eight dimensions can be summarized into two synthetic indices: the first four compose the "physical component", and the last four compose the "mental component" [5]. An additional one-item measure of self-evaluated change, from a year ago, in health status is also available. The raw scores are linearly translated into a scale with a minimum of 0 (worst condition) and a maximum of 100 (best condition), and the scores are evaluated using the Likert method for summed ratings. Also, the SF-36 dimensions are normalized into a scale ranging from 0 to 100.

Currently, to the author's knowledge, no studies establishing the clinically relevant change and clinically acceptable symptom state in the SF-36 score in patients who underwent rotator cuff repair have yet been published. Therefore, the current study is the first work aiming to find the MCID and PASS values for the SF-36 score after RCR. It was hypothesized that an MCID and PASS threshold could be identified in patients undergoing RCR.

2. Materials and Methods

A total of 46 patients (18 males and 28 females) of mean age 58.5 ± 12.9 years, all previously diagnosed with rotator cuff tears of any grade, were included in the study. Prior to their inclusion, the entire cohort underwent a comprehensive assessment involving general medical history, physical examination, and radiological examinations of the shoulder. The repair procedures for these patients were performed between September 2019 and September 2020 at Campus Bio-Medico in Rome.

The severity of the tears was evaluated through preoperative magnetic resonance imaging and clinical examinations, which were conducted by two orthopedic surgeons. The lesions were graded according to the Goutallier [6] grade and Patte [7] classifications. Prior to undergoing arthroscopic repair, all patients had undergone conservative treatment, which encompassed physiotherapy and a rehabilitation regimen. All patients underwent surgical repair, consistently carried out by a single experienced surgeon, who performed arthroscopic rotator cuff repairs for all 46 patients. All tears were successfully repaired. Patients with shoulder conditions unrelated to those requiring surgical intervention were excluded from the study. Each patient adhered to a standardized rehabilitation protocol.

During the initial four weeks post-surgery, an abduction sling pillow was employed to support the arm, allowing only active elbow extension and flexion. By the fifth week, supervised physiotherapy sessions were initiated, occurring one to three times per week, supplemented by exercises to be performed independently during the remaining time. Between the fifth and eighth weeks, the rehabilitation process introduced passive forward elevation, passive external rotation, and active assisted range of motion (ROM) exercises, gradually progressing to active ROM exercises. From the eighth to the tenth week, the rehabilitation regimen shifted towards strengthening the deltoid and scapular stabilizers, alongside concentric and eccentric exercise protocols targeting the rotator cuff muscles. The assessment of patients included administration of the SF-36 questionnaire during each evaluation time point.

The study was conducted according to the guidelines of the Declaration of Helsinki and was approved by the Institutional Review Board of Campus Bio-Medico University of Rome (COSMO study, Protocol number: 78/18 OSS ComEt CBM, 16/10/18).

2.1. Assessment Instruments

Six months after the rotator cuff repair, patients were presented with the following queries related to their satisfaction: "How do you feel after the surgery you have undergone?" and "Compared to a year ago, how do you feel?" to determine the MCID [8]. Two anchors were used to verify the consistency of results. For both questions, the available answers were "much worse", "a little worse", "equal", "a little better" and "much better". Patients who replied with "much worse", "a little worse" or "equal" were grouped into the "no-change" cohort, while patients who replied with "a little better" represented the "minimally improved" group. To calculate the PASS, patients were asked the question "Does shoulder pain affect the performance of your usual work activities (including domestic ones)?" at final evaluation. The potential answers were "Yes" or "No". An acceptable symptom state was attributed to patients who answered "No".

2.2. Statistical Analysis

A priori power analysis with an effect size of 0.71 (Cohen's d) [9], an alpha level of 0.05 (two-tailed), and a power of 0.80 revealed a minimum sample of 18 patients. Data normality for the SF-36 score and physical and mental dimensions of SF-36 at baseline and last follow-up using the Shapiro–Wilk test was established. Values at initial and final evaluations were compared using the Wilcoxon Signed Rank Test. The threshold for statistical significance was established at 0.05. SPSS version 26 for Windows (SPSS Inc., Chicago, IL, USA) was exploited for all statistical analyses.

The MCIDs for the SF-36 were estimated using a variety of anchor approaches and distribution-based methods. The following distribution-based tools were applied: 0.5 Standard Deviation (0.5 SD), the Standard Error of Measurement (SEM), and the Minimum Detectable Change (MDC). The 0.5 SD is correlated to effect size (0.5 SD is a median effect). The MDC correlates with the smallest variation above the measurement error with a confidence interval, while the SEM is the smallest variation above the measurement error (usually 95% confidence). For the present statistical analysis, Cronbach's alpha was applied as the measure of the reliability of the SF-36 in determining the SEM and MDC. The surgical satisfaction questionnaire was administered to patients for use as an anchor. Receiver Operating Characteristic (ROC) curves were exploited to determine the variation in SF-36 cut-off with maximized sensitivity and specificity. The Area Under the Curve (AUC) is considered the standard measure to assess the accuracy. It ranges in value from 0.5 (no better than chance) to 1.0 (perfect discrimination). Values of AUC less than 0.5 were considered not valid, and values of AUC less than 0.7 were considered not acceptable [10]. The MCID was also assessed via the Mean Change in SF-36 from initial evaluation (prior to intervention) to follow-up after the surgical procedure in patients who reported an improvement in surgical satisfaction. The pain questionnaire was used to calculate the PASS of SF-36. The 75th percentile of patients' cumulative percentage curve who self-assessed their symptom state to be satisfying was used to determine the PASS values of the SF-36 (patients who responded "No" at the pain questionnaire) and the point on the ROC curve, for which the threshold was calculated via the Youden index.

3. Results

Non-normal distribution of the SF-36 at initial screening and final evaluation was assessed using the Shapiro–Wilk test ($p < 0.05$).

At the initial evaluation, the average SF-36 score was 52.7 ± 17.2 (range 17.8–85.5) (0% floor and ceiling effects). At six months, the mean SF-36 score was 81.8 ± 14.6, ranging from 25.1 to 95.1 (0% floor and ceiling effects). A statistically relevant mean variation between initial and final evaluations was determined ($p < 0.001$). At baseline, the average physical component of the SF-36 score was 53.5 ± 17.8, ranging from 22.8 to 84.4 (0% floor and ceiling effects). At final follow-up, the mean physical component of the SF-36 score was 83.6 ± 17.6, ranging from 27.9 to 98.8 (0% floor and ceiling effects). A statistically significant mean variation between initial and final evaluations was found ($p < 0.001$).

At baseline, the average mental component of the SF-36 score was 65.6 ± 22.2 (range 16.9–95.5) (0% floor and ceiling effects). Six months post-operatively, the mean mental component of the SF-36 score was 84.1 ± 15, ranging from 28.6 to 98.8 (0% floor and ceiling effects). A statistically significant mean variation between initial and final screenings was assessed ($p < 0.001$).

The internal consistency reliability for the total, physical, and mental dimensions of the SF-36 was high ($\alpha = 0.9$) (Table 1).

Table 1. Summary of total, physical, and mental dimensions of the SF-36 score at baseline and six months' follow-up.

Score	Baseline Follow-Up			6-Month Follow-Up		
	Mean ± SD	Minimum	Maximum	Mean ± SD	Minimum	Maximum
Total SF-36	52.7 ± 17.2	17.8	85.5	81.8 ± 14.6	25.1	95.1
Physical SF-36	53.5 ± 17.8	22.8	84.4	83.6 ± 17.6	27.9	98.8
Mental SF-36	65.6 ± 22.2	16.9	95.5	84.1 ± 15	28.6	98.8

SF-36, 36-item short-form health survey questionnaire; SD, standard deviation.

3.1. Total, Physical, and Mental Components of SF-36

MCID estimates for the SF-36 for patients who underwent RCR ranged from 3.5 to 23.1. The following MCIDs with distribution-based approaches were computed: an MCID of 7.6 (0.5 SD) with a medium effect size (ES = 0.5); an MCID of 3.5 (SEM) with an internal consistency reliability of 0.9; an MCID of 9.6 (MDC) at the 95% confidence level (Table 2).

Table 2. MCID of SF-36 and dimensions of SF-36 in patients who underwent rotator cuff repair.

Score	0.5 SD	SEM	MDC	ROC (AUC)	Mean Change
Total SF-36	7.6	3.5	9.6	8.2 (0.8)	23.1
Physical SF-36	9.6	5.6	15.4	4.8 (0.9)	32.5
Mental SF-36	9.1	5.9	16.4	12 (0.6)	18.1

SF-36, 36-item short-form health survey questionnaire; SD, standard deviation; SEM, standard error of measurement; MDC, minimum detectable change; ROC, receiver operating characteristic; AUC, area under the curve.

3.2. MCID of Physical Dimension of SF-36

MCID estimates for the physical dimension of the SF-36 for patients who underwent RCR ranged from 5.6 to 32.5. The following MCIDs with distribution-based approaches were computed: an MCID of 9.6 (0.5 SD) with a medium effect size (ES = 0.5); an MCID of 5.6 (SEM) with an internal consistency reliability of 0.9; an MCID of 15.4 (MDC) at the 95% confidence level (Table 2).

3.3. MCID of Mental Dimension of SF-36

MCID estimates for the physical dimension of the SF-36 for patients who underwent RCR ranged from 5.9 to 18.1. The following MCIDs with distribution-based approaches were computed: an MCID of 9.1 (0.5 SD) with a medium effect size (ES = 0.5); an MCID of 5.9 (SEM) with an internal consistency reliability of 0.9; an MCID of 16.4 (MDC) at the 95% confidence level (Table 2).

3.4. PASS Values of SF-36

The SF-36 score with a PASS value of 81.9 had the highest levels of sensitivity and specificity. With the 75th percentile approach, 90.6 was the threshold. The PASS values of the physical dimension of the SF-36 were 88.3 and 94.5, using ROC and 75th percentile tools, respectively. The PASS values of the mental component of the SF-36 were 82 and 94.4, using ROC and 75th percentile approaches, respectively. All of these ROC calculations show high instrument responsiveness (AUC = 0.9, AUC = 0.9, and AUC = 0.8) (Table 3).

Table 3. PASS of SF-36 and dimensions of SF-36 in patients who underwent rotator cuff repair.

Score	ROC (AUC)	75th Percentile
Total SF-36	81.9 (0.9)	90.6
Physical SF-36	88.3 (0.9)	94.5
Mental SF-36	82 (0.8)	94.4

SF-36, 36-item short-form health survey questionnaire; ROC, receiver operating characteristic; AUC, area under the curve.

4. Discussion

The main finding of this article is that an improvement of 23.1 in the SF-36 score after a rotator cuff repair shows that patients' health improved in a way that is clinically significant. If 81.9 or more is attained in the SF-36 score after surgical repair, the majority of patients will find the symptom state satisfying.

A consistent technique for assessing patients' mental and physical health was created with the SF-36 survey. The clinical responsiveness of this questionnaire has been previously assessed by several authors [11–14]. However, MCIDs or PASS estimations for individuals with shoulder pathology have only been reported by a small number of authors. MCIDs and PASS have been reported in relation to several clinical scores, other than the SF-36, for patients who underwent RCR [15–21]. Among those, Cvetanovich and colleagues [18] provided essential insights into the MCID, substantial clinical benefit (SCB), and PASS thresholds in the context of individuals undergoing arthroscopic rotator cuff repair. Specifically, their study indicated that the corresponding threshold values for the ASES score were 11.1 for MCID, 17.5 for SCB, and 86.7 for PASS. Also, Tashjian et al. stated that a change at least of 4.3 in the SST score from pre-operative to post-operative time points corresponds to a minimal clinical improved in the patient [22]. At the same time, there have been several publications determining the MCID values in different surgical settings, such as total knee replacement, total hip replacement, and hip arthroscopic surgery [23–29]; however, no studies have yet evaluated the MCID and PASS of the SF-36 for patients undergoing RCR.

In the current literature, MCID estimates ranged between 3.3 and 24.9 for the SF-36. In the present study, the MCID for the SF-36 ranged from 3.5 to 23.1. It has been reported that a legitimate MCID should be at least bigger than the SEM value and depict how significant the patient believes the improvement (or worsening) to be [30]. Furthermore, as reported by Stipancic et al. [31], a useful MCID should be greater than the MDC. Therefore, the MCIDs calculated with the ROC method were useless because they were less than the MDC values [32–34]. Furthermore, since the AUC of the mental dimension of the SF-36 was less than 0.7, the MC method seems to be the most reliable in quantifying MCID values.

The MCID cut-offs of the total, physical, and mental dimensions of the SF-36 for patients who underwent RCR were 23.1, 32.5, and 18.1. These findings suggest that a variation greater than 9.6 for the SF-36, 15.4 for the physical dimension of the SF-36, and 16.4 for the mental dimension of the SF-36 (the MDC value) demonstrates that the change is not likely the result of random variation, while a change larger than 23.1 for the SF-36, 32.5 for the physical dimension of the SF-36, and 18.1 for the mental dimension of the SF-36 (the MCID values) reflects a clinically relevant variation.

The PASS for the SF-36 has not previously been estimated in any orthopedic study. This is the first paper in which the PASS for the SF-36 was calculated for patients who underwent RCR. The total SF-36 cut-offs were 81.9 (AUC = 0.9) with the ROC tool and 90.6 with the 75th percentile approach. The PASS values of SF-36′s physical dimension were 88.3 (AUC = 0.9) and 94.5, while for the mental dimension they were 82 (AUC = 0.8) and 94.4, using the ROC and 75th percentile methods, respectively. Given the high value of

AUC, the ROC tool appears to be the most accurate. Therefore, the PASS values of the total, physical, and mental dimensions of the SF-36 for patients who underwent RCR were 81.9, 88.3, and 82.

This study relies on several points of strength. This the first article that calculated the MCID and the PASS values of the SF-36 in patients who underwent RCR. Secondly, the MCID and PASS cut-offs were only determined using ad hoc techniques. Furthermore, both distribution and anchor approaches were exploited to establish the MCID, and to verify the consistency of results, two anchors were used to quantify the MCID.

Nonetheless, the current work also presents some weaknesses. The MCID and PASS were computed from baseline to a post-operative evaluation occurring only six months after the intervention and therefore cannot deliver long-term objective data. We have partially addressed this point of vulnerability by taking into consideration the long-term findings. These findings provide minimal evidence of alteration in SF-36 scores beyond the initial six-month period subsequent to RCR, extending up to a duration of 2 years. It is possible that the MCID thresholds may vary according to the different timing of the follow-up evaluation. The power analysis ascertained the adequacy of the enrolled patient count; nonetheless, it was grounded in a more substantial effect size than what was observed. Within this domain, it is customary to employ larger participant cohorts in published studies, and the limited patient population under evaluation in this review introduces the possibility of inherent bias.

5. Conclusions

The hypothesis of the current study was that MCID and PASS for patients undergoing RCR could be identified. A 23.1 improvement in the SF-36 score after RCR indicates that patients have achieved a clinically relevant amelioration in their health status. If 81.9 or more is attained in the SF-36 score after surgical repair, the majority of patients will consider their symptom state satisfactory.

Author Contributions: Conceptualization, U.G.L. and S.D.S.; methodology, B.B. and A.L.; software, I.P.; validation, U.G.L.; formal analysis, B.B. and A.L.; investigation, B.B. and A.L.; data curation, I.P., B.B. and A.L.; writing—original draft preparation, B.B. and A.L.; writing—review and editing, S.D.S.; visualization, V.D.; supervision, U.G.L.; project administration, V.D. All authors have read and agreed to the published version of the manuscript.

Funding: This research received no external funding.

Institutional Review Board Statement: The study was conducted according to the guidelines of the Declaration of Helsinki and approved by the Institutional Review Board of Campus Bio-Medico University of Rome (COSMO study, Protocol number: 78/18 OSS ComEt CBM, 16/10/18). The study was developed following Good Clinical Practice (GCP) guidelines.

Informed Consent Statement: The study was submitted to and approved by the ethics committee of "Campus Bio Medico" of Rome. All patients gave written consent to participate in the study.

Data Availability Statement: The data presented in this study are available on request from the corresponding author.

Conflicts of Interest: Professor Umile Giuseppe Longo is a guest Editor of the special issue of the Journal of Clinical Medicine. The rest of the authors declare that they have no conflicts of interest.

References

1. Angst, F.; Schwyzer, H.K.; Aeschlimann, A.; Simmen, B.R.; Goldhahn, J. Measures of adult shoulder function: Disabilities of the Arm, Shoulder, and Hand Questionnaire (DASH) and its short version (QuickDASH), Shoulder Pain and Disability Index (SPADI), American Shoulder and Elbow Surgeons (ASES) Society standardized shoulder assessment form, Constant (Murley) Score (CS), Simple Shoulder Test (SST), Oxford Shoulder Score (OSS), Shoulder Disability Questionnaire (SDQ), and Western Ontario Shoulder Instability Index (WOSI). *Arthritis Care Res.* **2011**, *63* (Suppl. S11), S174–S188. [CrossRef]
2. Jaeschke, R.; Singer, J.; Guyatt, G.H. Measurement of health status. Ascertaining the minimal clinically important difference. *Control Clin. Trials* **1989**, *10*, 407–415. [CrossRef] [PubMed]

3. Tubach, F.; Ravaud, P.; Baron, G.; Falissard, B.; Logeart, I.; Bellamy, N.; Bombardier, C.; Felson, D.; Hochberg, M.; van der Heijde, D.; et al. Evaluation of clinically relevant states in patient reported outcomes in knee and hip osteoarthritis: The patient acceptable symptom state. *Ann. Rheum. Dis.* **2005**, *64*, 34–37. [CrossRef]
4. Lins, L.; Carvalho, F.M. SF-36 total score as a single measure of health-related quality of life: Scoping review. *SAGE Open Med.* **2016**, *4*, 2050312116671725. [CrossRef] [PubMed]
5. Laucis, N.C.; Hays, R.D.; Bhattacharyya, T. Scoring the SF-36 in Orthopaedics: A Brief Guide. *J. Bone Jt. Surg. Am.* **2015**, *97*, 1628–1634. [CrossRef]
6. Somerson, J.S.; Hsu, J.E.; Gorbaty, J.D.; Gee, A.O. Classifications in Brief: Goutallier Classification of Fatty Infiltration of the Rotator Cuff Musculature. *Clin. Orthop. Relat. Res.* **2016**, *474*, 1328–1332. [CrossRef]
7. Lädermann, A.; Burkhart, S.S.; Hoffmeyer, P.; Neyton, L.; Collin, P.; Yates, E.; Denard, P.J. Classification of full-thickness rotator cuff lesions: A review. *EFORT Open Rev.* **2016**, *1*, 420–430. [CrossRef]
8. Tubach, F.; Ravaud, P.; Beaton, D.; Boers, M.; Bombardier, C.; Felson, D.T.; van der Heijde, D.; Wells, G.; Dougados, M. Minimal clinically important improvement and patient acceptable symptom state for subjective outcome measures in rheumatic disorders. *J. Rheumatol.* **2007**, *34*, 1188–1193.
9. Angst, F.; Goldhahn, J.; Drerup, S.; Aeschlimann, A.; Schwyzer, H.K.; Simmen, B.R. Responsiveness of six outcome assessment instruments in total shoulder arthroplasty. *Arthritis Rheum.* **2008**, *59*, 391–398. [CrossRef]
10. Hanley, J.A. The robustness of the "binormal" assumptions used in fitting ROC curves. *Med. Decis. Mak.* **1988**, *8*, 197–203. [CrossRef]
11. MacDermid, J.C.; Drosdowech, D.; Faber, K. Responsiveness of self-report scales in patients recovering from rotator cuff surgery. *J. Shoulder Elb. Surg.* **2006**, *15*, 407–414. [CrossRef]
12. Wang, W.; Zhang, C.; Cui, L.; Xie, Q.Y.; Jia, Z.Y.; Zheng, W. Reliability, validity and responsiveness of the Chinese version of the Rotator Cuff Quality of Life Index (RC-QOL) in patients with rotator cuff disorders. *PLoS ONE* **2018**, *13*, e0206347. [CrossRef] [PubMed]
13. Diniz Lopes, A.; Ciconelli, R.M.; Carrera, E.F.; Griffin, S.; Faloppa, F.; Baldy dos Reis, F. Comparison of the responsiveness of the Brazilian version of the Western Ontario Rotator Cuff Index (WORC) with DASH, UCLA and SF-36 in patients with rotator cuff disorders. *Clin. Exp. Rheumatol.* **2009**, *27*, 758–764. [PubMed]
14. Böhm, T.D.; Kirschner, S.; Köhler, M.; Wollmerstedt, N.; Walther, M.; Matzer, M.; Faller, H.; König, A. The German Short Musculoskeletal Function Assessment questionnaire: Reliability, validity, responsiveness, and comparison with the Short Form 36 and Constant score--a prospective evaluation of patients undergoing repair for rotator cuff tear. *Rheumatol. Int.* **2005**, *25*, 86–93. [CrossRef]
15. Kukkonen, J.; Kauko, T.; Vahlberg, T.; Joukainen, A.; Aärimaa, V. Investigating minimal clinically important difference for Constant score in patients undergoing rotator cuff surgery. *J. Shoulder Elb. Surg.* **2013**, *22*, 1650–1655. [CrossRef] [PubMed]
16. Tashjian, R.Z.; Deloach, J.; Green, A.; Porucznik, C.A.; Powell, A.P. Minimal clinically important differences in ASES and simple shoulder test scores after nonoperative treatment of rotator cuff disease. *J. Bone Jt. Surg. Am.* **2010**, *92*, 296–303. [CrossRef] [PubMed]
17. Tashjian, R.Z.; Deloach, J.; Porucznik, C.A.; Powell, A.P. Minimal clinically important differences (MCID) and patient acceptable symptomatic state (PASS) for visual analog scales (VAS) measuring pain in patients treated for rotator cuff disease. *J. Shoulder Elb. Surg.* **2009**, *18*, 927–932. [CrossRef]
18. Cvetanovich, G.L.; Gowd, A.K.; Liu, J.N.; Nwachukwu, B.U.; Cabarcas, B.C.; Cole, B.J.; Forsythe, B.; Romeo, A.A.; Verma, N.N. Establishing clinically significant outcome after arthroscopic rotator cuff repair. *J. Shoulder Elb. Surg.* **2019**, *28*, 939–948. [CrossRef]
19. Haunschild, E.D.; Gilat, R.; Fu, M.C.; Tauro, T.; Huddleston, H.P.; Yanke, A.B.; Forsythe, B.; Verma, N.N.; Cole, B.J. Establishing the Minimal Clinically Important Difference, Patient Acceptable Symptomatic State, and Substantial Clinical Benefit of the PROMIS Upper Extremity Questionnaire After Rotator Cuff Repair. *Am. J. Sports Med.* **2020**, *48*, 3439–3446. [CrossRef]
20. Xu, S.; Chen, J.Y.; Lie, H.M.E.; Hao, Y.; Lie, D.T.T. Minimal Clinically Important Difference of Oxford, Constant, and UCLA shoulder score for arthroscopic rotator cuff repair. *J. Orthop.* **2020**, *19*, 21–27. [CrossRef]
21. Kim, D.M.; Kim, T.H.; Kholinne, E.; Park, J.H.; Shin, M.J.; Kim, H.; Park, D.; Jeon, I.H.; Koh, K.H. Minimal Clinically Important Difference, Substantial Clinical Benefit, and Patient Acceptable Symptomatic State After Arthroscopic Rotator Cuff Repair. *Am. J. Sports Med.* **2020**, *48*, 2650–2659. [CrossRef] [PubMed]
22. Tashjian, R. Editorial Commentary: The Alphabet Soup of Understanding Clinical Shoulder Research: MCID (Minimal Clinically Important Difference), PASS (Patient Acceptable Symptomatic State), SCB (Substantial Clinical Benefit), and Now... MOI (Maximal Outcome Improvement). *Arthroscopy* **2020**, *36*, 1811–1812. [CrossRef] [PubMed]
23. Escobar, A.; Quintana, J.M.; Bilbao, A.; Aróstegui, I.; Lafuente, I.; Vidaurreta, I. Responsiveness and clinically important differences for the WOMAC and SF-36 after total knee replacement. *Osteoarthr. Cartil.* **2007**, *15*, 273–280. [CrossRef] [PubMed]
24. Quintana, J.M.; Escobar, A.; Bilbao, A.; Arostegui, I.; Lafuente, I.; Vidaurreta, I. Responsiveness and clinically important differences for the WOMAC and SF-36 after hip joint replacement. *Osteoarthr. Cartil.* **2005**, *13*, 1076–1083. [CrossRef] [PubMed]
25. Keurentjes, J.C.; Van Tol, F.R.; Fiocco, M.; Schoones, J.W.; Nelissen, R.G. Minimal clinically important differences in health-related quality of life after total hip or knee replacement: A systematic review. *Bone Jt. Res.* **2012**, *1*, 71–77. [CrossRef] [PubMed]

26. Bin Abd Razak, H.R.; Tan, C.S.; Chen, Y.J.; Pang, H.N.; Tay, K.J.; Chin, P.L.; Chia, S.L.; Lo, N.N.; Yeo, S.J. Age and Preoperative Knee Society Score Are Significant Predictors of Outcomes Among Asians Following Total Knee Arthroplasty. *J. Bone Jt. Surg. Am.* **2016**, *98*, 735–741. [CrossRef] [PubMed]
27. Teo, B.J.X.; Koh, J.S.B.; Jiang, L.; Allen, J.C.; Yeo, S.J.; Howe, T.S. Association of the 36-Item Short Form Health Survey Physical Component Summary Score With Patient Satisfaction and Improvement 2 Years After Total Knee Arthroplasty. *JAMA Netw. Open* **2019**, *2*, e190062. [CrossRef] [PubMed]
28. Carton, P.; Filan, D. Defining the Minimal Clinically Important Difference in Athletes Undergoing Arthroscopic Correction of Sports-Related Femoroacetabular Impingement: The Percentage of Possible Improvement. *Orthop. J. Sports Med.* **2020**, *8*, 2325967119894747. [CrossRef]
29. Yeo, M.G.H.; Goh, G.S.; Chen, J.Y.; Lo, N.N.; Yeo, S.J.; Liow, M.H.L. Are Oxford Hip Score and Western Ontario and McMaster Universities Osteoarthritis Index Useful Predictors of Clinical Meaningful Improvement and Satisfaction After Total Hip Arthroplasty? *J. Arthroplast.* **2020**, *35*, 2458–2464. [CrossRef]
30. Copay, A.G.; Glassman, S.D.; Subach, B.R.; Berven, S.; Schuler, T.C.; Carreon, L.Y. Minimum clinically important difference in lumbar spine surgery patients: A choice of methods using the Oswestry Disability Index, Medical Outcomes Study questionnaire Short Form 36, and pain scales. *Spine J.* **2008**, *8*, 968–974. [CrossRef]
31. Stipancic, K.L.; Yunusova, Y.; Berry, J.D.; Green, J.R. Minimally Detectable Change and Minimal Clinically Important Difference of a Decline in Sentence Intelligibility and Speaking Rate for Individuals With Amyotrophic Lateral Sclerosis. *J. Speech Lang. Hear. Res.* **2018**, *61*, 2757–2771. [CrossRef] [PubMed]
32. Çelik, D.; Çoban, Ö.; Kılıçoğlu, Ö. Minimal clinically important difference of commonly used hip-, knee-, foot-, and ankle-specific questionnaires: A systematic review. *J. Clin. Epidemiol.* **2019**, *113*, 44–57. [CrossRef] [PubMed]
33. MacKay, C.; Clements, N.; Wong, R.; Davis, A.M. A systematic review of estimates of the minimal clinically important difference and patient acceptable symptom state of the Western Ontario and McMaster Universities Osteoarthritis Index in patients who underwent total hip and total knee replacement. *Osteoarthr. Cartil.* **2019**, *27*, 1408–1419. [CrossRef] [PubMed]
34. Maredupaka, S.; Meshram, P.; Chatte, M.; Kim, W.H.; Kim, T.K. Minimal clinically important difference of commonly used patient-reported outcome measures in total knee arthroplasty: Review of terminologies, methods and proposed values. *Knee Surg. Relat. Res.* **2020**, *32*, 19. [CrossRef]

Journal of
Clinical Medicine

MDPI

Article

Classification and Incidence of Heterotopic Ossifications in Relation to NSAID Prophylaxis after Elbow Trauma

Diane Leyder [1,*], Stefan Döbele [1,2], Christian Konrads [2,3], Tina Histing [1], Cornelius S. Fischer [1], Marc-Daniel Ahrend [1] and Patrick Ziegler [2,4]

1 Department of Traumatology and Reconstructive Surgery, BG Unfallklinik Tübingen, Eberhard Karls University of Tübingen, 72074 Tübingen, Germany
2 Medical Faculty, University of Tübingen, 72074 Tübingen, Germany; christian.konrads@gmail.com (C.K.)
3 Department of Orthopaedics and Traumatology, Helios Hanseatic Hospital Stralsund, 18435 Stralsund, Germany
4 Department of Orthopaedics and Trauma Surgery, Klinik Gut, 7500 St. Moritz, Switzerland
* Correspondence: dleyder@bgu-tuebingen.de; Tel.: +49-7071-606-3954

Abstract: Heterotopic ossification (HO) after elbow trauma can be responsible for significant motion restrictions. The study's primary aim was to develop a new X-ray-based classification for HO of the elbow. This retrospective study analyzed elbow injury radiographs from 138 patients aged 6–85 years (mean 45.9 ± 18) who underwent operative treatment. The new classification was applied at 6 weeks, 12 weeks, and 6 months postoperatively. The severity of HO was graded from 0 to 4 and localization was defined as r (radial), p (posterior), u (ulnar) or a (anterior) by two observers. The patients were categorized based on injury location and use of non-steroidal anti-inflammatory drugs (NSAIDs) for HO prophylaxis. The correlations between the generated data sets were analyzed using Chi-square tests (χ^2) with a significance level of $p < 0.05$. The inter- and intraobserver reliability was assessed using Cohen's Kappa. In 50.7% of the evaluated X-rays, the formation of HO could be detected after 12 weeks, and in 60% after 6 months. The analysis showed a significant correlation between the injury's location and the HO's location after 12 weeks ($p = 0.003$). The use of an NSAID prophylaxis did not show a significant correlation with the severity of HO. The classification showed nearly perfect inter- ($\kappa = 0.951$, $p < 0.001$) and intrareliability ($\kappa = 0.946$, $p < 0.001$) according to the criteria of Landis and Koch. Based on the presented classification, the dimension and localization of HO in the X-ray image can be described in more detail compared to previously established classifications and, thus, can increase the comparability of results across studies.

Keywords: elbow trauma; heterotopic ossifications; classification; stiff elbow; HO prophylaxis

1. Introduction

Heterotopic ossifications (HO) can occur as a complication after elbow injuries. New lamellar bone is formed in soft tissue, which can occur due to an accompanying inflammatory reaction to a trauma [1–3]. Severe forms in the joint area can lead to considerable functional restrictions [4–6].

The prevalence of HO shows a wide variance of 10–20% after traumatic brain or spinal cord injury; 20% after forearm fractures; up to 52% after femur fractures, total hip arthroplasty or acetabular fractures; and up to 60% after severe burns [7]. HO's pathophysiology is not yet fully understood, but tissues prone to HO have excessive inflammatory responses to injury. Recent studies show mesenchymal stem cells and their increased bone morphogenic protein (BMP) activity lead to vascular proliferation and bone formation in HO [8].

The incidence of HO at the elbow joint varies significantly. Douglas et al. reported that 35% of patients required surgical intervention of more severe ossifications after distal intra-articular humerus fractures, while 26% needed the same procedure after elbow dislocation fractures [9]. Liu et al. conducted a systematic review involving over 2000 patients and found that 10% developed radiologically visible HO after total elbow arthroplasty [10]. Wahl et al. investigated the incidence and location of HO after elbow injuries and found that almost all patients developed HO, which could be statistically linked to the injury site [11].

There are various ways to clinically measure the stiffness of an elbow joint. Morrey's scoring system divides elbow stiffness into three categories: intrinsic, extrinsic, and combined stiffness [12]. Another scoring system, developed by Kay, classifies elbow stiffness based on the involved anatomical structure, which could be soft tissue, bony stiffness, or a combination of both [13]. In Kay's system, HO refers to bony or combined elbow stiffness.

To radiologically define elbow stiffness and determine the presence of HO, two classifications are used: Brooker's classification was originally designed for the hip joint and is based on X-ray images in one plane. It presents five categories, from the absence of HO to a bone brace [14]. The Hastings and Graham classification was designed for the elbow. In this classification, a distinction between the presence or absence of HO is made with focus on the functional limitations [15]. However, neither of these classifications describe the localization of ossifications. This is especially relevant in the case of elbow joint ossifications, as their location can be used to predict the extent of elbow functional limitation and can also aid in planning revision surgery or radiotherapy. Furthermore, utilizing standardized nomenclature can offer several benefits for the assessment of HO and may assist in optimizing and standardizing therapy options [11].

Therapeutic options for expired HO are limited to surgical excision, which often has unsatisfactory results [16,17]. Early detection and prevention of HO are therefore the priority. Non-steroidal anti-inflammatory drugs (NSAIDs) and radiation are most commonly used to prevent HO [18]. Several systematic reviews and meta-analyses have shown that NSAIDs can prevent heterotopic ossification (HO), particularly after total hip arthroplasty [19–21]. NSAIDs work by inhibiting the differentiation of mesenchymal stem cells, which are the precursor cells of osteoblasts, and by reducing the production of pro-inflammatory prostaglandins [22]. However, despite ongoing research, there is significant inconsistency in the available evidence regarding their effectiveness after elbow trauma [22–24].

This study presents a novel radiographic classification system that precisely describes the degree and location of HO, thereby improving objectivity and functional assessment. We aim to demonstrate, based on our hypothesis, that HO occurs at the same site as the primary injury. Additionally, we aim to establish a correlation between the use of ossification prophylaxis and the development of HO in our cohort.

2. Materials and Methods

2.1. Patient Collective and Study Design

This retrospective study was approved by the local ethics committee. The records of 273 patients with surgically treated elbow injuries between January 2015 and December 2020 were analyzed based on inclusion and exclusion criteria. Of the total number of patients considered, 135 were disqualified due to reasons such as spinal cord injury (n = 1), traumatic brain injury (n = 15), receiving treatment from a different hospital (n = 11), infections (n = 1), or a follow-up period of less than 12 weeks (n = 135). Consequently, 138 patients were deemed eligible and included in the study. Clinical and radiological follow-up exams were conducted at 6 (n = 138) and 12 weeks (n = 138) as well as 6 months (n = 75) post-surgery. The flowchart of patients is shown in Figure 1.

2.2. Radiographic Assessment

The analysis of the radiographs was performed initially by a single person using the Xero Universal Viewer software Version 1.0.0.R812 (Xero Universal Viewer, Agfa Health Care Corp. Greenville, SC, USA). For this purpose, standard X-rays of the elbow in two planes (anterior to posterior (AP) and lateral radiographs) were performed two days after the initial surgery. Any preexisting bone avulsions, osteophytes, or ossifications were defined. Follow-up radiographs were realized after six and twelve weeks (n = 138), as well as after six months (n = 75). After one year, two surgeons in different stages of training reviewed all X-ray images again, blinded to the first interpretation. The images were then analyzed and classified according to the following classification based on the apparent HO.

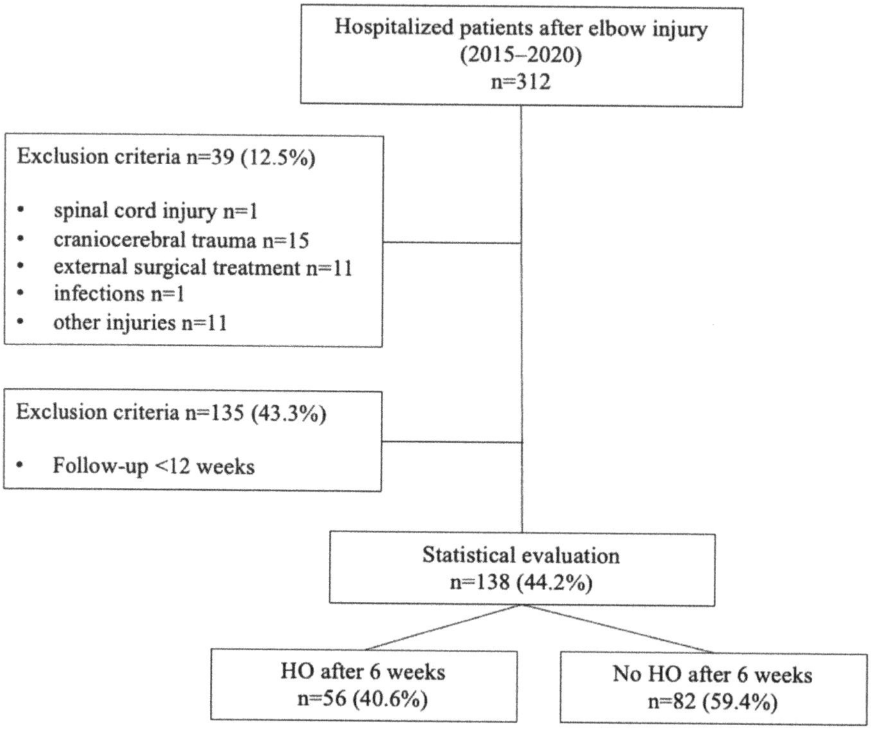

Figure 1. Flowchart of analyzed patients.

2.3. *Classification*

For the new classification (Table 1), the localization of HO was defined as follows: radial (r), posterior (p), ulnar (u), and anterior (a). The severity of HO was graded from 0 (no ossifications) to 4 (synostosis). The largest visible HO in terms of length was considered. The classification was determined as follows: 0 means no HO; 1 means visible HO, which is smaller in size than the diameter of the radial head; 2 means a larger diameter than the radial head; 3 indicates a brace formation from the humerus to the forearm; and 4 describes the synostosis radio-ulnar.

Table 1. HO classification.

	Severity	Localization
Absence of HO	0	
<∅ radial head	1	r, p, u, a
>∅ radial head	2	r, p, u, a
Brace formation	3	r, p, u, a
Synostosis radio-ulnar	4	

r—radial, p—posterior, u—ulnar, a—anterior.

Since regular radiographs usually do not have a reference sphere, the diameter of the radial head was defined as the cutoff size between severity grades one and two. Thus, the classification is independent of a reference sphere, and the size ratio from the examined elbow is included. Examples of each grade of severity are shown in Figures 2–5.

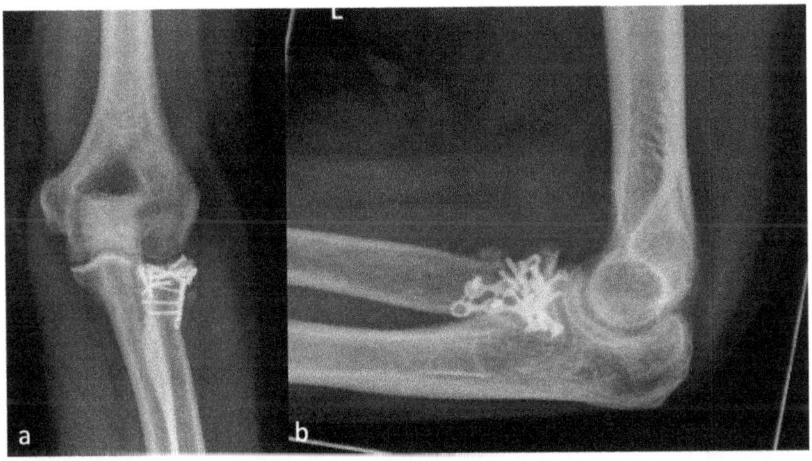

Figure 2. (**a**) The AP and (**b**) the lateral X-ray with a radial HO smaller than the diameter of the radial head, which represents an HO 1 r.

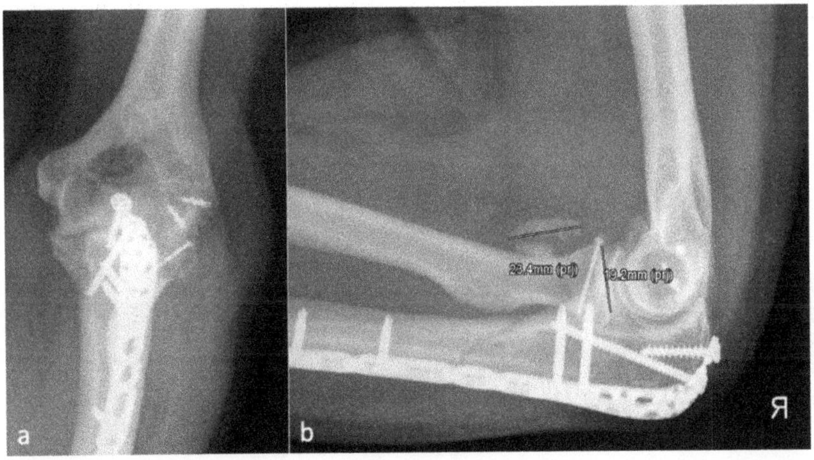

Figure 3. (**a**) shows the AP and (**b**) shows the lateral X-ray with an anterior HO (23.4 mm) which is larger than the diameter of the radial head (19.2 mm) and represents an HO 2a.

2.4. Further Parameters

The study included a total of 138 patients who were categorized based on their age, sex, and type of injury. We verified the use of ossification prophylaxis by checking the hospital medication records and discharge letters. Ossification prophylaxis was considered to be taken if prescribed for 14 days. Additionally, we determined the location of each injury through a review of the initial X-ray and MRI images taken after the injury.

Five categories of injury were defined:

- Lateral: radial head fracture, LCL tear, lateral condyle fractures of the humerus.
- Ventral: Coronoid fractures.

- Medial: MCL tear, medial condyle fractures of the humerus.
- Dorsal: Olecranon fractures.
- Multilateral: Distal humerus fractures (AO C 1–3), Monteggia fractures, Monteggia-like-lesions, LCL, and MCL rupture at the same time.

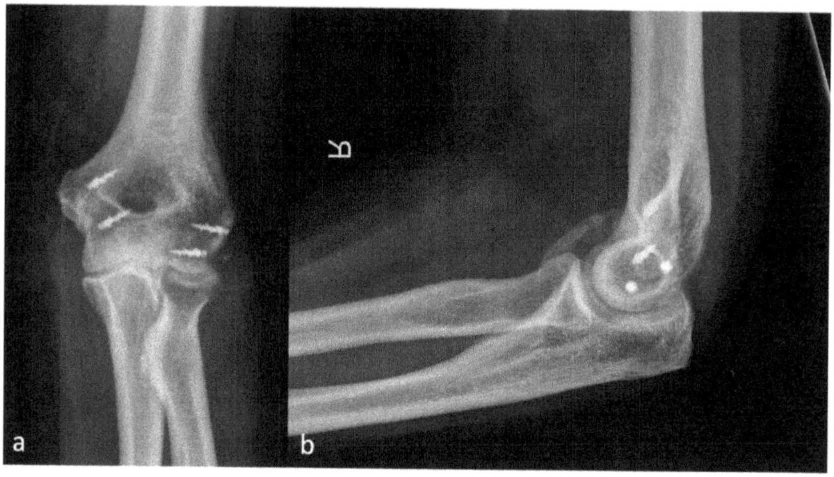

Figure 4. (**a**) shows the AP and (**b**) shows the lateral X-ray with an anterior HO forming a brace from the humerus to the forearm, representing an HO 3a.

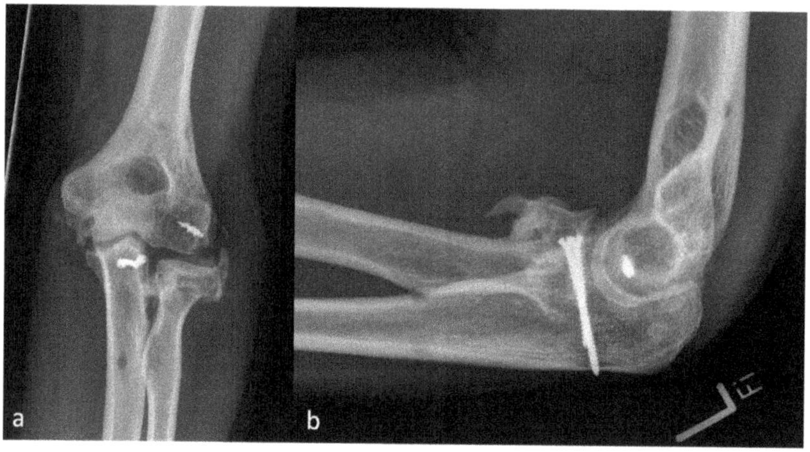

Figure 5. (**a**) shows the AP and (**b**) shows the lateral X-ray with a brace formation radio-ulnar and represents an HO 4.

2.5. Statistical Analysis

Descriptive statistics were performed using absolute and relative frequencies (n (%)) or mean ± standard deviation. The incidence of HO was measured after 6 weeks, 12 weeks, and 6 months. The incidence of the injury location at the elbow and the injured structures was calculated.

This study used Cohen's Kappa coefficient κ to determine the intra- and interobserver reliability of HO severity and localization. Based on Landis and Koch's method, values were categorized as ≤0 (no agreement), 0.01–0.20 (none to slight), 0.21–0.40 (fair), 0.41–0.60 (moderate), 0.61–0.80 (substantial), and 0.81–1.00 (almost perfect agreement) [25].

To examine the correlation between HO severity and the use of ossification prophylaxis and between the location of the injury and the developed HO, four-field tables were implemented to present the frequencies of the associations, and significance calculation was performed using the Chi-squared test (χ^2). A significance level with $p < 0.05$ was defined. The statistical analysis of the collected data was performed using a statistical program (SPSS Statistics®, IBM, Armonk, NY, USA, version 28).

3. Results

3.1. Descriptive Statistics

Among the 138 patients included, 73 (52.9%) were male patients and 65 (47.1%) were female patients. The mean age at trauma was 45.9 ± 18 years (6 to 85 years). The radial head was affected in 61 (44.2%), the coronoid in 36 (26.1%), the olecranon in 22 (15.9%), and the distal humerus in 34 (24.6%) cases. Regarding ligament injuries, the lateral collateral ligament was considered unstable in 33 (23.9%), the lateral and medial collateral ligaments in 38 (27.5%), and the medial collateral ligament alone in three cases (2.2%).

Of the total number of patients under observation, it was noted that a majority of them (102 (73.9%) patients) received prophylaxis for ossification for 14 days, while the remaining 36 (26.1%) did not receive any NSAID prophylaxis. Among the patients who received prophylaxis, 47 (33.9%) were given Indomethacin (100 mg/day), 53 (64.5%) were given Ibuprofen (800–1800 mg/day), and 1 patient each was given Etoricoxib (90 mg/day) or Celecoxib (400 mg/day).

The incidence of HO after 6 weeks (5.8 ± 2.3 weeks) was 40.6% (Grade I 35.5%, Grade II 4.3% and Grade III 0.7%), after 12 weeks (16.4 ± 10.9 weeks) 50.7% (Grade I 41.3%, Grade II 6.5% and Grade III 2.9%), and after 6 months (29.9 ± 10.9 weeks) 60.0% (Grade I 40.0%, Grade II 12.0%, Grade III 2.7%, and Grade IV 5.3%). Details regarding the location and severity of HO are summarized in Table 2.

Table 2. HO Incidence after 6 and 12 weeks and 6 months.

	HO Incidence (%)	Severity Incidence of HO (%)		Location Incidence of HO (%)	
		HO Grade		HO Localization	
6 weeks	56 (40.6)	0 1 2 3	82 (59.4) 49 (35.5) 6 (4.3) 1 (0.7)	r p u a	18 (32.1) 6 (10.7) 11 (19.6) 21 (37.5)
12 weeks	70 (50.7)	0 1 2 3	68 (49.3) 57 (41.3) 9 (6.5) 4 (2.9)	r p u a	15 (26.8) 5 (8.9) 12 (21.4) 23 (41.1)
6 months	45 (60.0)	0 1 2 3 4	30 (40.0) 30 (40.0) 9 (12.0) 2 (2.7) 4 (5.3)	r p u a	10 (31.3) 1 (3.1) 5 (15.6) 16 (50.0)

r—radial, p—posterior, u—ulnar, a—anterior.

3.2. Relationship between Injury Localization and the Localization of HO

The study found a significant relation (χ^2 = 28.3, p = 0.005) between the location of the injury (lateral, posterior, medial, anterior, multilateral) and the location of a HO (radial, posterior, ulnar, anterior) after 6 weeks. The correlation remained significant even after 12 weeks (χ^2 = 25.5, p = 0.003). However, after 6 months, the correlation was no longer significant (χ^2 = 9.1, p = 0.421).

3.3. Correlation between the Application of Ossification Prophylaxis and the Severity of HO

After 6 weeks, we found no significant correlation ($\chi^2 = 1.0$, $p = 0.797$) between the severity of HO and the application of ossification prophylaxis. The same results were observed after 12 weeks ($\chi^2 = 0.9$, $p = 0.876$) and after 6 months ($\chi^2 = 5.5$, $p = 0.244$) in this cohort. After comparing the two most commonly used methods for preventing ossification, Indomethacin and Ibuprofen, it was found that there was no significant correlation between the severity of HO and the medication taken. This was observed after 6 weeks ($\chi^2 = 4.7$, $p = 0.197$), after 12 weeks ($\chi^2 = 0.9$, $p = 0.819$), and after 6 months ($\chi^2 = 4.3$, $p = 0.363$).

3.4. Intra- and Interobserver Reliability

The level of agreement between raters (interreliability) was found to be almost perfect in both the categorization of the severe gradient ($\kappa = 0.951$, $p < 0.001$) and the classification of the localization of HO ($\kappa = 0.953$, $p < 0.001$). Similarly, the level of agreement within the same rater (intrareliability) was almost perfect for both the severity grade ($\kappa = 0.946$, $p < 0.001$) and the localization ($\kappa = 0.949$, $p < 0.001$) of HO.

4. Discussion

In the present study, the formation and extent of ossifications at the elbow joint were investigated based on radiological signs concerning the injury pattern and localization. Based on the analyzed data, a classification for HO at the elbow was developed. The goal of the present study was to simplify and standardize the classification of HO around the elbow.

4.1. Classification

The aim was to develop a classification that is easy to apply. The severity of HO was divided into five different categories (0–4). Furthermore, the localization of the ossification could be documented by the addition of the letters (anterior, posterior, radial, ulnar). This differs from existing classifications, such as the Hastings and Graham classification, which focuses predominantly on the restriction of movement [15]. The inter- and intrareliability for both the severity level and localization of HO classification was almost perfect. Whether the proposed classification can be easily applied in a clinical daily routine needs to be shown by further studies and regular applications in clinical practice.

4.2. Incidences of HO

The incidence of HO after surgically treated elbow injuries in our collective (up to 60%) is much higher than the average values presented in the literature. For example, Herman et al. described an incidence of 28.7% after surgically treated elbow fractures [26]. Foruria et al. studied distal humerus fractures that were primarily treated via osteosynthesis; here, 42% showed HO at 12 weeks [27]. Hong et al. also examined elbows for HO with a follow-up of 6 months. No ossification prophylaxis was taken by the 124 patients and only 30% showed HO [28].

The higher incidences found in this study may be due to the fact that all the patients included in the study underwent surgical treatment. This could have triggered a second inflammatory response in addition to the trauma, potentially leading to an increase in HO [3]. Also, our cohort may be biased as it does not equally represent conservatively and surgically treated elbow injuries.

Radiographic controls were conducted 6 and 12 weeks after the surgery, and out of the 138 patients who were scheduled for these follow-ups, only 75 patients returned for the examination after 6 months. It is possible that patients with mild symptoms did not return for control, unlike those with more persistent complaints. Given the nature of our data collection, it is important to note that our findings are limited to the analysis of elbow injuries that have been treated surgically and may still exhibit residual symptoms. This means that any conclusions drawn from our study should be considered within the context of this specific population.

Furthermore, a significant correlation was found between the location of the injury and the localization of HO at 6 and 12 weeks. However, after 6 months, this correlation was no longer significant. It was observed that HO is formed laterally in 30% of cases and anteriorly in 50%. This suggests that in most elbow injuries, the ventral capsule might also be affected, and the associated inflammatory reaction might trigger the formation of HO. The same findings were described by Wahl et al., one of the very few studies that also investigated elbow injuries and the localization of HO [11].

4.3. Prophylaxis of HO

In the study, the analysis did not show any significant difference in the development of HO between the groups with NSAID prophylaxis and the one without. The literature on the subject presents contradictory statements. For instance, Bochat et al. examined 153 patients who underwent surgical treatment for elbow injuries, with 78 patients receiving ossification prophylaxis and 72 not receiving it. Yet, again, no significant difference was found between the two groups [22]. In a randomized controlled trial published in 2023, there was no significant difference in the development of HO one year after elbow injury between patients who received Indomethacin or a placebo [23]. On the other hand, Costopoulos et al. found a significant difference in the development of radioulnar synostosis after distal biceps tendon refixation between patients who received Indomethacin and those who did not receive prophylaxis [29]. The available data on the efficacy of ossification prophylaxis (NSAIDs) are still subject to controversy. Conclusions drawn for HO prophylaxis in the context of surgical treatment of the hip joint cannot be transferred to the elbow without further examinations based on our research and the data collected. Despite several studies other studies showing no benefit of this treatment, its use remains widespread [30]. Further randomized studies are necessary to clarify the situation and determine whether the benefits outweigh the risks.

4.4. Limitations

This study aimed to propose a new classification system for elbow heterotopic ossifications and accepted its limitations, utilizing a retrospective study design.

One other limitation is that in some cases, the accurate classification of the location of the injury was difficult due to unclear transitions. Patients with multiple bone injuries or injuries in combination with a ligamentous lesion were classified as multilateral injuries. Predominantly in elbow dislocations with or without fractures, the main injury could not be clearly defined [31]. The classification of the injury was performed depending on the available diagnostic data. X-rays and CT were performed on most patients after the accident. An MRI examination, however, was only performed if there was a clinical suspicion of an additional ligamentous or cartilage lesion. This may lead to some undocumented ligament injuries.

In the future, for these cases, a prospective analysis of elbow injuries with a standardized diagnostic pathway including MRI might be an option to include these cases more correctly in the data evaluation. Furthermore, only the radiological presence or absence of HO was considered. The correlation with the functional limitation should be investigated further to determine the clinical significance more precisely. Also, due to the retrospective study design used to analyze the effectiveness of ossification prophylaxis, it was not possible to evaluate the treatment duration and patient compliance, even though it was recommended for 14 days. Therefore, further prospective studies are needed to explore the prophylaxis's efficacy more closely. And finally, it must be pointed out once again that these were exclusively surgically treated patients and that the examined injuries represented a very heterogeneous collective.

5. Conclusions

The current scientific understanding of the formation of HO in the elbow joint after trauma is still incomplete. Nevertheless, our classification system can easily categorize

HO, making it easier to evaluate. Hopefully, this study can assist in collecting more data and conducting further research to gain a better understanding of HO. This is crucial in reducing the risk of movement restrictions and revision surgery due to HO and providing patients with evidence-based prevention and treatment.

Author Contributions: Conceptualization, C.K.; Formal analysis, D.L.; Investigation, D.L.; Resources, C.S.F.; Writing—original draft, D.L.; Writing—review & editing, M.-D.A. and P.Z.; Supervision, S.D., T.H. and P.Z.; Project administration, P.Z. All authors have read and agreed to the published version of the manuscript.

Funding: This research received no external funding.

Institutional Review Board Statement: The study was conducted in accordance with the Declaration of Helsinki and approved by the Ethical Committee Eberhard Karls University (Tübingen Trial registration: 020/2021BO2, 2 February 2021).

Informed Consent Statement: Informed consent was obtained from all subjects involved in the study.

Data Availability Statement: The data presented in this study are available on request from the corresponding author.

Conflicts of Interest: The authors declare no conflicts of interest.

References

1. Matsuo, K.; Chavez, R.D.; Barruet, E.; Hsiao, E.C. Inflammation in Fibrodysplasia Ossificans Progressiva and Other Forms of Heterotopic Ossification. *Curr. Osteoporos. Rep.* **2019**, *17*, 387–394. [CrossRef]
2. Ramirez, D.M.; Ramirez, M.R.; Reginato, A.M.; Medici, D. Molecular and cellular mechanisms of heterotopic ossification. *Histol. Histopathol.* **2014**, *29*, 1281–1285. [CrossRef] [PubMed]
3. Evans, K.N.; Forsberg, J.A.; Potter, B.K.; Hawksworth, J.S.; Brown, T.S.; Andersen, R.; Dunne, J.R.; Tadaki, D.; Elster, E.A. Inflammatory cytokine and chemokine expression is associated with heterotopic ossification in high-energy penetrating war injuries. *J. Orthop. Trauma* **2012**, *26*, e204–e213. [CrossRef] [PubMed]
4. Vasileiadis, G.I.; Ramazanian, T.; Kamaci, S.; Bachman, D.R.; Park, S.E.; Thaveepunsan, S.; Fitzsimmons, J.S.; O'Driscoll, S.W. Loss of pronation-supination in patients with heterotopic ossification around the elbow. *J. Shoulder Elb. Surg.* **2019**, *28*, 1406–1410. [CrossRef] [PubMed]
5. Wiggers, J.K.; Helmerhorst, G.T.; Brouwer, K.M.; Niekel, M.C.; Nunez, F.; Ring, D. Injury complexity factors predict heterotopic ossification restricting motion after elbow trauma. *Clin. Orthop. Relat. Res.* **2014**, *472*, 2162–2167. [CrossRef] [PubMed]
6. Veltman, E.S.; Lindenhovius, A.L.; Kloen, P. Improvements in elbow motion after resection of heterotopic bone: A systematic review. *Strateg. Trauma Limb Reconstr.* **2014**, *9*, 65–71. [CrossRef]
7. Dey, D.; Wheatley, B.M.; Cholok, D.; Agarwal, S.; Yu, P.B.; Levi, B.; Davis, T.A. The traumatic bone: Trauma-induced heterotopic ossification. *Transl. Res.* **2017**, *186*, 95–111. [CrossRef] [PubMed]
8. Lin, L.; Shen, Q.; Leng, H.; Duan, X.; Fu, X.; Yu, C. Synergistic inhibition of endochondral bone formation by silencing Hif1α and Runx2 in trauma-induced heterotopic ossification. *Mol. Ther.* **2011**, *19*, 1426–1432. [CrossRef]
9. Douglas, K.; Cannada, L.K.; Archer, K.R.; Dean, D.B.; Lee, S.; Obremskey, W. Incidence and risk factors of heterotopic ossification following major elbow trauma. *Orthopedics* **2012**, *35*, e815–e822. [CrossRef]
10. Liu, E.Y.; Hildebrand, A.; Horner, N.S.; Athwal, G.S.; Khan, M.; Alolabi, B. Heterotopic ossification after total elbow arthroplasty: A systematic review. *J. Shoulder Elb. Surg.* **2019**, *28*, 587–595. [CrossRef]
11. Wahl, E.P.; Casey, P.M.; Risoli, T.; Green, C.L.; Richard, M.J.; Ruch, D.S. Heterotopic ossification formation after fractures about the elbow. *Eur. J. Orthop. Surg. Traumatol.* **2021**, *31*, 1061–1067. [CrossRef]
12. Morrey, B.F. The posttraumatic stiff elbow. *Clin. Orthop. Relat. Res.* **2005**, *431*, 26–35.
13. Masci, G.; Cazzato, G.; Milano, G.; Ciolli, G.; Malerba, G.; Perisano, C.; Greco, T.; Osvaldo, P.; Maccauro, G.; Liuzza, F. The stiff elbow: Current concepts. *Orthop. Rev.* **2020**, *12* (Suppl. 1), 8661. [CrossRef] [PubMed]
14. Brooker, A.F.; Bowerman, J.W.; Robinson, R.A.; Riley, L.H. Ectopic ossification following total hip replacement. Incidence and a method of classification. *J. Bone Jt. Surg. Am.* **1973**, *55*, 1629–1632. [CrossRef]
15. Hastings, H.; Graham, T.J. The classification and treatment of heterotopic ossification about the elbow and forearm. *Hand Clin.* **1994**, *10*, 417–437. [CrossRef] [PubMed]
16. Koh, K.H.; Lim, T.K.; Lee, H.I.; Park, M.J. Surgical treatment of elbow stiffness caused by post-traumatic heterotopic ossification. *J. Shoulder Elb. Surg.* **2013**, *22* (Suppl. 1), 1128–1134. [CrossRef] [PubMed]
17. Salazar, D.; Golz, A.; Israel, H.; Marra, G. Heterotopic ossification of the elbow treated with surgical resection: Risk factors, bony ankylosis, and complications. *Clin. Orthop. Relat. Res.* **2014**, *472*, 2269–2275. [CrossRef] [PubMed]
18. Sun, Y.; Cai, J.; Li, F.; Liu, S.; Ruan, H.; Fan, C. The efficacy of celecoxib in preventing heterotopic ossification recurrence after open arthrolysis for post-traumatic elbow stiffness in adults. *J. Shoulder Elb. Surg.* **2015**, *24*, 1735–1740. [CrossRef]

19. Joice, M.; Vasileiadis, G.I.; Amanatullah, D.F. Non-steroidal anti-inflammatory drugs for heterotopic ossification prophylaxis after total hip arthroplasty: A systematic review and meta-analysis. *Bone Jt. J.* **2018**, *100*, 915–922. [CrossRef]
20. Kan, S.L.; Yang, B.; Ning, G.Z.; Chen, L.X.; Li, Y.L.; Gao, S.J.; Chen, X.Y.; Sun, J.C.; Feng, S.Q. Nonsteroidal Anti-inflammatory Drugs as Prophylaxis for Heterotopic Ossification after Total Hip Arthroplasty: A Systematic Review and Meta-Analysis. *Medicine* **2015**, *94*, e828. [CrossRef]
21. Ma, R.; Chen, G.H.; Zhao, L.J.; Zhai, X.C. Efficacy of naproxen prophylaxis for the prevention of heterotopic ossification after hip surgery: A meta-analysis. *J. Orthop. Surg. Res.* **2018**, *13*, 48. [CrossRef] [PubMed]
22. Bochat, K.; Mattin, A.C.; Ricciardo, B.J. The efficacy of nonsteroidal anti-inflammatories in the prevention of heterotopic ossification following elbow trauma surgery. *JSES Int.* **2021**, *5*, 793–796. [CrossRef] [PubMed]
23. Atwan, Y.; Abdulla, I.; Grewal, R.; Faber, K.J.; King, G.J.W.; Athwal, G.S. Indomethacin for heterotopic ossification prophylaxis following surgical treatment of elbow trauma: A randomized controlled trial. *J. Shoulder Elb. Surg.* **2023**, *32*, 1242–1248. [CrossRef] [PubMed]
24. Li, F.; Mao, D.; Pan, X.; Zhang, X.; Mi, J.; Rui, Y. Celecoxib cannot inhibit the progression of initiated traumatic heterotopic ossification. *J. Shoulder Elb. Surg.* **2019**, *28*, 2379–2385. [CrossRef] [PubMed]
25. Landis, J.R.; Koch, G.G. The measurement of observer agreement for categorical data. *Biometrics* **1977**, *33*, 159–174. [CrossRef]
26. Herman, Z.J.; Edelman, D.G.; Ilyas, A.M. Heterotopic Ossification After Elbow Fractures. *Orthopedics* **2021**, *44*, 10–16. [CrossRef]
27. Foruria, A.M.; Lawrence, T.M.; Augustin, S.; Morrey, B.F.; Sanchez-Sotelo, J. Heterotopic ossification after surgery for distal humeral fractures. *Bone Jt. J.* **2014**, *96*, 1681–1687. [CrossRef]
28. Hong, C.C.; Nashi, N.; Hey, H.W.; Chee, Y.H.; Murphy, D. Clinically relevant heterotopic ossification after elbow fracture surgery: A risk factors study. *Orthop. Traumatol. Surg. Res.* **2015**, *101*, 209–213. [CrossRef]
29. Costopoulos, C.L.; Abboud, J.A.; Ramsey, M.L.; Getz, C.L.; Sholder, D.S.; Taras, J.P.; Huttman, D.; Lazarus, M.D. The use of indomethacin in the prevention of postoperative radioulnar synostosis after distal biceps repair. *J. Shoulder Elb. Surg.* **2017**, *26*, 295–298. [CrossRef]
30. Winkler, S.; Wagner, F.; Weber, M.; Matussek, J.; Craiovan, B.; Heers, G.; Springorum, H.R.; Grifka, J.; Renkawitz, T. Current therapeutic strategies of heterotopic ossification—A survey amongst orthopaedic and trauma departments in Germany. *BMC Musculoskelet. Disord.* **2015**, *16*, 313. [CrossRef]
31. O'Driscoll, S.W.; Morrey, B.F.; Korinek, S.; An, K.N. Elbow subluxation and dislocation. A spectrum of instability. *Clin. Orthop. Relat. Res.* **1992**, *280*, 186–197.

Journal of
Clinical Medicine

MDPI

Case Report

Tackling Kinesiophobia in Chronic Shoulder Pain: A Case Report on the Combined Effect of Pain Education and Whole-Body Cryostimulation

Angelo Alito [1], Mariachiara Elisabetta Cifalinò [2], Jacopo Maria Fontana [2,*], Federica Verme [2], Paolo Piterà [3] and Paolo Capodaglio [2,4]

1 Department of Biomedical, Dental Sciences and Morphological and Functional Images, University of Messina, 98125 Messina, Italy; alitoa@unime.it
2 Research Laboratory in Biomechanics, Rehabilitation and Ergonomics, IRCCS, Istituto Auxologico Italiano, San Giuseppe Hospital, Piancavallo, 28824 Verbania, Italy; mchiara.cif@gmail.com (M.E.C.); f.verme@auxologico.it (F.V.); p.capodaglio@auxologico.it (P.C.)
3 Department of Clinical and Biological Sciences, University of Turin, Orbassano, 10043 Torino, Italy; p.pitera@auxologico.it
4 Department of Surgical Sciences, Physical and Rehabilitation Medicine, University of Torino, 10121 Torino, Italy
* Correspondence: j.fontana@auxologico.it

Abstract: Background: Chronic shoulder pain may cause significant functional disability and reduced psychosocial well-being. Detailed Case Description: In this case, we propose the use of pain neuroscience education and whole-body cryostimulation (WBC) to treat a 64-year-old woman with severe functional limitations and chronic right shoulder pain. The aim was to overcome kinesiophobia and improve her motor function, autonomy, and quality of life. Functional and clinical assessments were conducted at admission, discharge, and at a one-month follow-up via phone call. The patient's global health, shoulder function, and quality of life showed improvement during hospitalisation and were maintained after one month. Discussion: Pain education is crucial in managing chronic shoulder pain, especially in addressing kinesiophobia and promoting positive patient outcomes. In this context, WBC was used as a supplementary treatment to traditional pain relief and exercise tolerance therapies. This can help individuals to participate more actively in their rehabilitation process, ultimately promoting functional recovery and an improved quality of life. Conclusion: The combination of cryostimulation, tailored physical exercises, pain education, manual therapy, and psychological support created a synergistic effect that addressed both the physical and psychological aspects of pain and kinesiophobia.

Keywords: chronic shoulder pain; kinesiophobia; pain education; rehabilitation; whole-body cryostimulation

1. Introduction

Chronic pain is recognised as a condition lasting beyond the physiological healing period persisting or recurring for more than 3–6 months [1,2].

Shoulder pain is a common musculoskeletal condition accounting for approximately 1.3% of all general practice presentations [3,4]. Incidence and prevalence rates tend to increase with age (degenerative processes), in women (anatomical, biomechanical and hormonal factors), in lower socioeconomic groups (reduced access to healthcare structures, physically demanding occupations), and in psychologically stressed populations (somatisation and increased pain sensitivity) [5,6].

Identifying the cause of a shoulder pain can be difficult due to the large number of structures such as bones, ligaments, tendons, and bursae that can be involved in the onset of pain or dysfunction [7]. In addition, these parts must maintain bone congruence, which guarantees dynamic stability for all the range of motion (ROM) [8].

Patients with chronic shoulder pain often experience significant functional disability and reduced psychosocial well-being, and to best manage the shoulder condition, accurate diagnosis is essential, and clinical assessment and imaging studies must be carefully considered [9].

Many shoulder pathologies such as rotator cuff, long head biceps tendon or labrum lesions, bursitis, adhesive capsulitis, osteoarthritis, acromioclavicular joint disease, or instability can present with similar symptoms (e.g., pain, weakness, ROM limitation) [10]. As a result, there is a wide range of treatment options, from conservative management, including activity modification, systemic (e.g., analgesics or anti-inflammatories) or local (e.g., intraarticular injections) medications, to manual treatment, therapeutic exercise, and surgical treatment [8,11].

Indeed, many biopsychosocial factors have been linked to the chronicisation of pain, leading to anxiety, poorer recovery and quality of life (QoL), and sometimes to pain avoidance beliefs [12,13].

Kinesiophobia is an excessive, irrational, and disabling fear of movement or activity due to a sense of vulnerability to painful injury or re-injury and is often associated with avoidance behaviours such as altered motor patterns that may limit actual functional capacity [14,15].

To prevent physical damage, people learn to avoid movements and activities that they find painful and to adopt different or alternative behaviours [16,17].

This can lead to reduced shoulder range of motion and stiffness, potentially leading to further limitation of ROM and functionality, resulting in muscle weakness and disuse, deconditioning of normal movement and adoption of maladaptive motor patterns [14]. In addition, the maintenance of these symptoms can lead to psychological distress, which can exacerbate the perception of pain, perpetuating this vicious cycle, prolonging rehabilitation time, and limiting participation in therapeutic exercise and recovery [18].

Higher levels of fear-avoidance beliefs are associated with greater levels of motor impairment and disability, so communication between healthcare providers and patients, including education, disease information, treatment goals and reassurance, may also help recovery and play an important role in rehabilitation outcomes [19–21].

In this context, pain neuroscience education (PNE), as an ongoing process based on an understanding of pain physiology, sensitisation, and its role in chronic pain, can represent a core strategy in pain management, aiming to reconceptualise the understanding of pain as less threatening [22–24].

Several studies have shown that PNE can reduce pain, disability, catastrophising and kinesiophobia in the short to medium term [25,26] and there are different types of treatment modalities, such as individual education through oral dialogue, group treatments, and information through the provision of a booklet and/or printed materials [27].

The literature has shown that the most effective intervention is the individual interview, which allows treatment to be specific and individualised for each patient, creating a patient–clinician therapeutic alliance that improves treatment outcomes [28].

Furthermore, the multifaceted interactions and consequences of chronic pain and kinesiophobia require a multidisciplinary approach that addresses the complex interplay between physical, psychological, and social factors [14,29].

Because of its rapid effect on overall well-being by modulating pain and improving mobility, whole-body cryostimulation (WBC) has been used as an adjuvant therapy in several conditions and could play an important role in the treatment of chronic pain [30–32]. The effects of cryostimulation have been shown to be beneficial in several systems such as haematological, metabolic, and musculoskeletal, as well as with an anti-inflammatory effect, in post-exercise and post-traumatic recovery, pain and physical performance, and in psychological aspects [30,33]. This treatment consists of repeated daily sessions of 2–3 min in which the whole body is exposed to extremely low temperatures (−110 to −140 °C) in cryogenic chambers with the aim of reducing inflammation and vasoconstriction, modulating pain transmission, and regulating the release of neurotransmitters [29].

The aim of this work is to provide evidence on the role of a multidisciplinary rehabilitation programme involving PNE and WBC in overcoming kinesiophobia and improving patients' motor function, autonomy, and quality of life.

This case report followed the CARE guidelines for case reports [34].

2. Detailed Case Description

A 64-year-old woman was admitted to the rehabilitation department of the Istituto Auxologico Italiano, Piancavallo (VB) in December 2023 with severe functional impotence of the right shoulder. She presented with a history of diabetes mellitus type 2, cervical and lumbar discopathy, and polyarthralgia. She also reported chronic low back pain with a previous lumbar microdiscectomy about twenty years ago and left knee pain with meniscopathy and patellofemoral chondropathy.

The impairment of the right shoulder started in the last months of 2021 with a progressive development of pain and functional limitations. She underwent an orthopaedic consultation which prescribed restriction of shoulder movements and physiotherapy, not recommending surgery. The patient started rehabilitation treatment based on physiotherapy and mild shoulder mobilisation with no clinical improvement. In January 2022, she underwent an MRI scan due to persistent pain. This revealed mild acromioclavicular arthrosis, severe tendinosis of the supraspinatus tendon with oedema and intratendinous microinjuries in the critical area, mild tendinosis of the infraspinatus tendon with a thin film of fluid in the subacromial deltoid bursa, and a mild effusion on the tendinous sheath of the long head of the biceps (Figure 1).

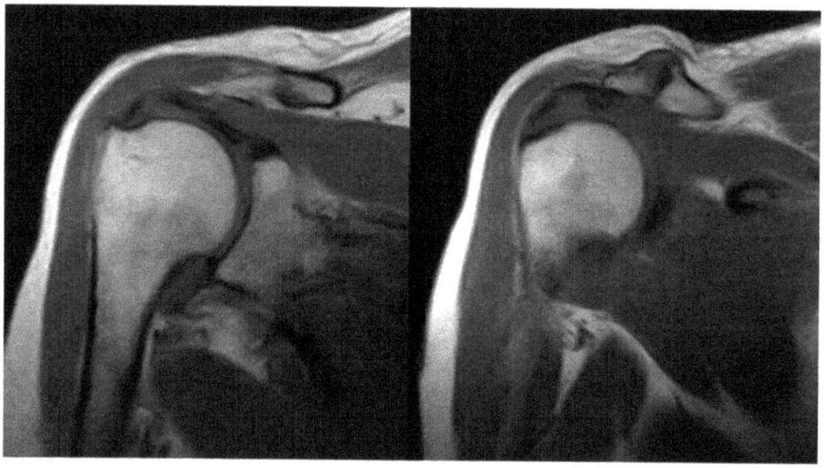

Figure 1. Shoulder MRI showing mild acromioclavicular arthrosis and severe supraspinatus tendinosis with intratendinous microinjuries and oedema.

Then, she underwent two cycles of physiotherapy, mainly physical therapy modalities (e.g., laser therapy, ultrasound therapy) with little clinical benefit. Meanwhile, she was taking NSAIDs to control the pain, and between June and July 2023 she underwent a cycle of three intraarticular injections of steroids with mild clinical benefit. The persistence and worsening of the pain led the patient to a progressive limitation of shoulder movements with the development of fear-avoidance behaviours until her admission to the S. Giuseppe Hospital of Piancavallo in December 2023.

At the first physiatric assessment, the patient presented with an autonomous normal gait, a swayback posture, severe antalgic limitation of active movements of the right shoulder with severe mid-range pain, reduced ROM, and significant kinesiophobia. There were no neurological symptoms (i.e., paraesthesia or sensory deficits).

At the physiotherapy assessment, the patient presented with her right arm in an antalgic position and expressed considerable concern about movement-related pain, treatment modality, and prognosis. She complained of persistent pain and increased use of her left arm to avoid painful movements and her autonomy with activities of daily living (ADLs) was very limited, often requiring assistance. Shoulder examination revealed severe antalgic ROM limitation, particularly in flexion, abduction, and internal rotation (NRS 10/10), combined with a fear of movement.

The patient underwent multidisciplinary treatment, including a dietary plan, physiotherapy sessions, and psychological support and, in addition, given the repeated failures of the previous approach about pain management, and given the absence of contraindications, the physicians suggested the implementation of WBC treatment.

The physiotherapy sessions focused on therapeutic exercise, manual therapy, and pain education, with the aim of restoring full range of motion and desensitising chronic pain. The rehabilitation program started with passive shoulder mobilisation in a pain-free ROM, progressed to an active/assisted modality with acceptable pain, then progressive isotonic exercises to gradually return to physiological movements. Finally, a progressive strength training program was implemented based on the patient's positive feedback.

Treatment sessions included individualised pain education through verbal interviews discussing the physiology of the pain system, the characteristics, purpose, and origin of acute and chronic pain, the mechanisms of pain chronicisation and the potential factors contributing to central sensitisation such as emotions, stress, illness, perception, pain cognition, and pain behaviour.

In addition, the patient performed five daily WBC sessions (2 min/−110 °C) in a cryochamber (Artic, CryoScience, Rome, Italy) with an optimal treatment adherence, subjective reduction in pain and satisfaction, and no adverse effects reported.

Functional and clinical assessments were performed at admission and discharge. Global function was assessed using the 6 min walk test (6MWT) [35], overall strength using the hand grip test (HGT) [36], and general well-being using the Psychological General Well-being Index (PGWBI) [37]. Shoulder evaluation was performed by measuring ROM with a goniometer, the Disabilities of the Arm, Shoulder and Hand (DASH) questionnaire [38], and the Shoulder Pain and Disability Index (SPADI) [39]. In addition, the Short-Form Health Survey 36 (SF-36) [40] was used to measure health-related quality of life (HR-QoL) and the Tampa Scale for Kinesiophobia (TSK) [41] to quantify fear of painful movement. During the hospital stay, the patient reported a subjective improvement in physical performance, shoulder movements, and a global reduction in pain. A global view of the assessments is provided in Table 1.

Table 1. Comprehensive admission and discharge assessments: A global view of functional and psychological well-being.

	Admission	Discharge
6MWT (m)	405	492
NRS (0–10)	10	3
HGT (kg)	RH 23.7 LH 19.2	RH 24.2 LH 19.6
PGWBI	50	75
Passive Right Shoulder ROM		
Flexion	120°	180°
Extension	25°	30°
Abduction	110°	180°
Internal Rotation	40°	100°
External Rotation	30°	35°

6MWT, 6 min walk test; HGT, hand grip strength test; LH, left hand; NRS, numerical rating scale; PGWBI, Psychological General Well-being Index; RH, right hand; ROM, range of motion.

The patient also underwent an X-ray exam of the right shoulder that showed no focal bone morpho-structural changes and mild evidence of acromioclavicular arthrosis (Figure 2) and an additional MRI scan that showed an osteo-fibrous sleeve of the acromion-clavicular joint with impingement of the tendon of the supraspinatus muscle with a full-thickness anterosuperior lesion. In addition, tendinosis of the tendon of the subscapularis muscle with bursitis was noted (Figure 3).

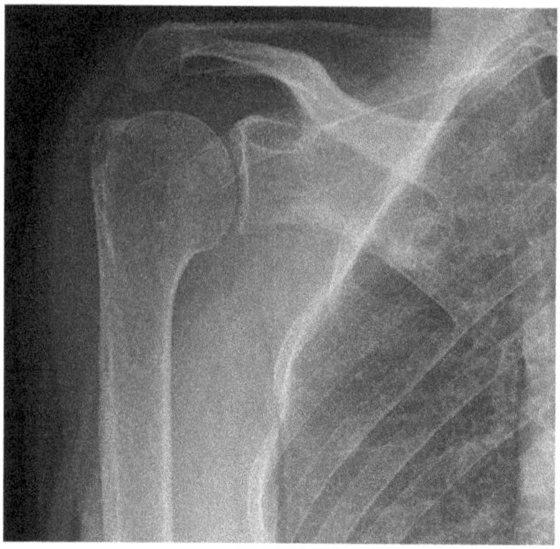

Figure 2. Radiograph of the right shoulder in extrarotation showing mild acromioclavicular arthrosis.

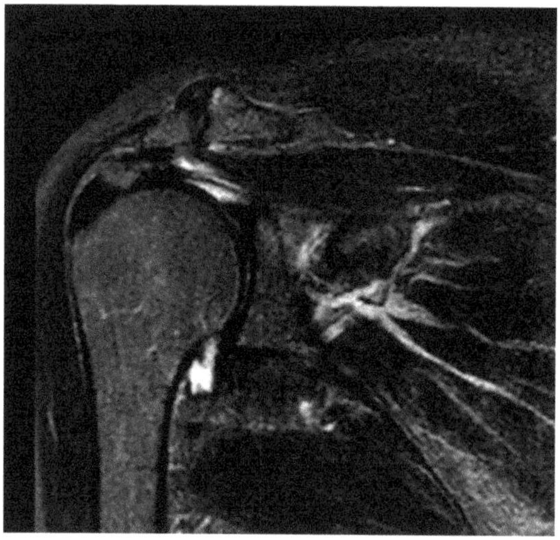

Figure 3. The pre-discharge MRI shows an osteofibrous sleeve of the acromion-clavicular joint with impingement of the supraspinatus tendon with a full-thickness anterosuperior lesion.

After discharge, a follow-up telephone call was made to inquire about general health, maintenance of results achieved during hospitalisation, and to re-complete the DASH, SPADI, TSK and SF-36. The patient reported that she returned to her normal lifestyle with an overall improvement in global health, shoulder function (Table 2), and quality of life (Table 3, Figure 4). A comprehensive timeline of clinical history and interventions is shown in Figure 5.

Table 2. Measure progress over time: Admission, discharge, and 1-month follow-up scales for comprehensive assessment of patient outcomes.

	Admission	Discharge	One-Month Follow-Up
DASH (%)	79.31	28.44	25.8
SPADI (%)			
Pain	84	42	14
Disability	90	63.7	11.3
Total SPADI Score	87.7	55.4	12.3
TSK			
Activity avoidance (6–24)	19	8	7
Somatic Focus (7–28)	18	9	7
Total TSK Score (13–52)	37	17	14

DASH, Disabilities of the Arm, Shoulder, and Hand questionnaire; SPADI, Shoulder Pain and Disability Index; TSK, Tampa Scale for Kinesiophobia.

Table 3. Tracking quality of life outcomes: SF-36 results at admission, discharge, and 1-month follow-up, providing insights into patient well-being across the healthcare continuum.

Score (%)	Admission	Discharge	One-Month Follow-Up
Physical functioning	35	70	70
Role limitations due to physical health	25	100	50
Role limitations due to emotional problems	33.3	100	100
Energy/fatigue	40	70	80
Emotional well-being	40	76	84
Social functioning	25	75	100
Physical pain	22.5	67.5	67.5
General health	50	60	65
Health Change	50	100	100

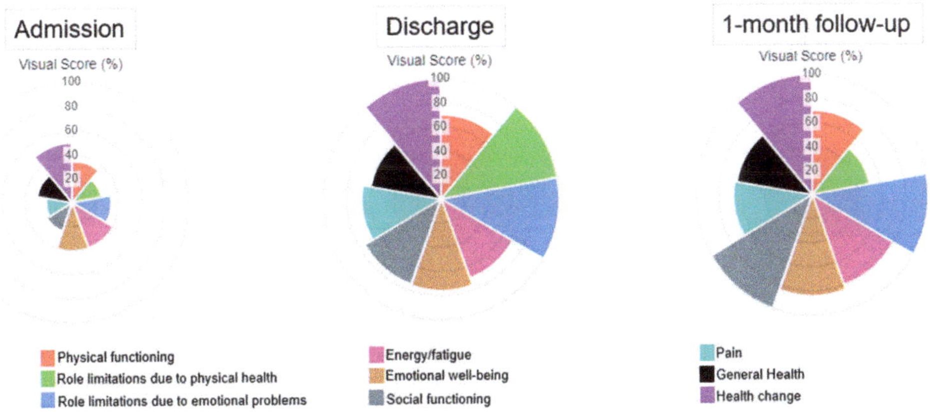

Figure 4. Visualising well-being: SF-36 graphical representation capturing dynamic changes in quality of life at admission, discharge and one-month follow-up; https://orthopowertools.com/SF36 (accessed on 26 January 2024).

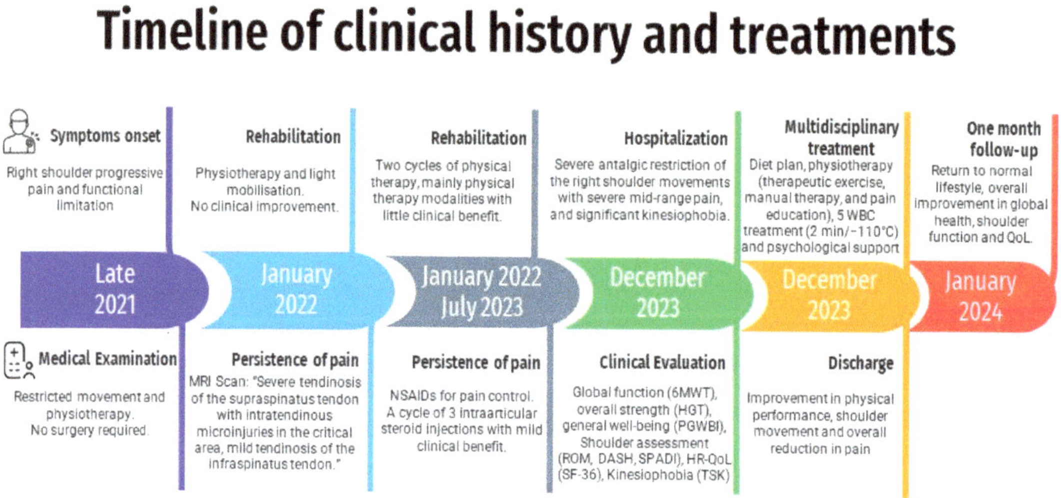

Figure 5. Reporting medical progress: A timeline of patient clinical history and interventions.

3. Discussion

Chronic pain is a disabling condition that affects millions of people worldwide, not only physically but also emotionally and psychologically [1,42]. As well as physical discomfort, it can lead to fear, anxiety, and avoidance behaviours [43]. As a result, kinesiophobia is a common problem among people experiencing chronic pain, with a significant impact on quality of life, leading to reduced mobility, muscle weakness, and even further pain and disability [44].

Understanding kinesiophobia is an important component of chronic pain management, as it can greatly affect a patient's motivation to comply with physical therapy and rehabilitation programs [18,45].

Healthcare providers can assist patients in overcoming their fears and gradually increasing their confidence in movement and exercise by addressing and educating them [46,47].

In this case study, the patient suffered from chronic shoulder pain for a few years, and the initial moderate pain and limitation of movement resulted in the patient consulting several medical specialists. The failure of repeated treatments and maintenance of pain led to a progressive reduction in shoulder use and function as well as mood.

Over time, the chronicisation of pain evolved into a significant level of kinesiophobia, with fear and hesitation to move the right shoulder or engage in any form of exercise, exacerbated by previous experiences of pain during physical activity.

The physiotherapist used a personalised approach, explaining the underlying mechanisms of pain and the importance of gradually challenging her fear of movement, addressing the patient's beliefs and gradually changing her perception of movement from a source of fear to a pathway to recovery.

To further address the patient's chronic shoulder limitation and pain, a WBC cycle was implemented in this multidisciplinary approach with the aim to facilitate the rehabilitation process.

Over time, this rehabilitation approach resulted in a quite complete resolution of symptoms and improvement in the patient's confidence in physical activity, regaining shoulder mobility and function even one month after discharge, with the patient maintaining most of the achieved improvements.

Interestingly, the psychological effects of using an innovative device may play a role in better adherence to rehabilitation treatment and the known effects of WBC on pain, especially in the short term, may have an adjunctive effect to physical therapy.

WBC has gained attention for its potential benefits in the management of chronic pain by inducing a systemic response, leading to various physiological and biochemical changes that can effectively modulate pain perception, reduce inflammatory markers, and improve overall pain tolerance [30,32]. It helps to reduce swelling and oedema in the affected area by inducing vasoconstriction, thus providing relief from pain and discomfort [48]. WBC may also exert local analgesic effects by reducing nerve transmission throughout the body, combined with increased endorphin concentration and norepinephrine production released from both peripheral nerve terminals and brain nuclei by sympathetic stimulation, ultimately reducing the perception of pain [49–51]. WBC also has significant psychosocial implications, as the release of endorphins and other neurotransmitters not only relieves pain but also plays a crucial role in reducing the psychological barriers associated with chronic pain, such as anxiety and depression [52,53].

In this context, WBC can serve as a complementary intervention to traditional pain relief and exercise tolerance therapies, enabling individuals to participate more actively in their rehabilitation process and ultimately promoting functional recovery and improved quality of life [30,54].

The results obtained in this patient are also consistent with the study by Ma and colleagues who compared physiotherapy modalities and joint mobilisation with the same treatments plus WBC in patients with shoulder adhesive capsulitis [50].

Pain education and support from healthcare professionals is essential to help people understand their active role in pain management, address common misconceptions and beliefs about kinesiophobia, reduce anxiety and develop a better attitude, and focus on the recovery process [22,55].

Studies suggest that factors such as pain catastrophising, kinesiophobia, and ineffective pain management methods play a crucial role in understanding the diversity of pain levels and physical functioning in people with chronic shoulder pain [56].

As a result, the importance of a biopsychosocial approach has been progressively emphasised, and recent approaches include therapeutic exercise, physiotherapy combined with adjuvant treatments (i.e., WBC), pharmacological pain management, and patient education [57].

Indeed, in this case study, the combination of cryostimulation with tailored physical exercises, pain education, manual therapy, and psychological support helped to create a synergistic effect that addressed both the physical and psychological aspects of pain and kinesiophobia.

However, there are some limitations to this case study, and the positive results must be interpreted with caution. Firstly, the lack of generalisability due to the nature of the study and the lack of a standardised protocol makes it difficult to establish causality or to determine the true significance of the observed results.

The patients' positive emotional involvement in the treatment and high level of satisfaction may have played a role in the observed global functional improvement, so a placebo effect cannot be excluded. In addition, the authors cannot determine the component of the rehabilitation program that may have played the most important role in the results.

To the best of our knowledge, this is the first case reporting on the effects of a multimodal approach, involving WBC and pain education in a case of kinesiophobia in chronic shoulder pain. Future research should further investigate the long-term efficacy and optimal dosage of this combined approach, as well as its application to different patient groups and clinical settings.

4. Conclusions

This case report illustrates the effectiveness of a multimodal approach with the integration of physical therapy, pain education, and WBC in the management of chronic shoulder pain, particularly in overcoming both the physiological and psychosocial aspects of kinesiophobia and facilitating medium-term recovery. The combined approach of WBC and PNE is a valid strategy for the treatment of kinesiophobia, highlighting the complementary and synergistic effects of these approaches in reducing fear-avoidance behaviours and improving pain coping mechanisms. The subjective experience of the patients, from very early sessions, is that WBC provides a rapid sense of well-being and reduces the perception of pain, leading to improved compliance with rehabilitation treatments and that the combined effects of pain education and pathways play an important role in improving the patients' health status.

Author Contributions: Conceptualisation, A.A. and F.V.; methodology, J.M.F. and P.C.; investigation, F.V. and M.E.C.; writing—original draft preparation, A.A., F.V., M.E.C. and P.P.; writing—review and editing, J.M.F. and P.C. All authors have read and agreed to the published version of the manuscript.

Funding: This work was supported by Italian Ministry of Health—Ricerca Corrente.

Institutional Review Board Statement: The study was conducted in accordance with the Declaration of Helsinki and approved by the Institutional Ethics Committee of Istituto Auxologico Italiano (protocol code 2021_05_18_14, approved 18 May 2021).

Informed Consent Statement: Written informed consent was obtained from the patient to publish this paper.

Data Availability Statement: The data presented in this study are available within the article.

Conflicts of Interest: The authors declare no conflicts of interest.

References

1. Raffaeli, W.; Tenti, M.; Corraro, A.; Malafoglia, V.; Ilari, S.; Balzani, E.; Bonci, A. Chronic Pain: What Does It Mean? A Review on the Use of the Term Chronic Pain in Clinical Practice. *J. Pain Res.* **2021**, *14*, 827–835. [CrossRef] [PubMed]
2. Treede, R.D.; Rief, W.; Barke, A.; Aziz, Q.; Bennett, M.I.; Benoliel, R.; Cohen, M.; Evers, S.; Finnerup, N.B.; First, M.B.; et al. A classification of chronic pain for ICD-11. *Pain* **2015**, *156*, 1003–1007. [CrossRef] [PubMed]
3. Ristori, D.; Miele, S.; Rossettini, G.; Monaldi, E.; Arceri, D.; Testa, M. Towards an integrated clinical framework for patient with shoulder pain. *Arch. Physiother.* **2018**, *8*, 7. [CrossRef] [PubMed]
4. Murphy, R.J.; Carr, A.J. Shoulder pain. *BMJ Clin. Evid.* **2010**, *2010*, 1107. [PubMed]
5. Greving, K.; Dorrestijn, O.; Winters, J.C.; Groenhof, F.; van der Meer, K.; Stevens, M.; Diercks, R.L. Incidence, prevalence, and consultation rates of shoulder complaints in general practice. *Scand. J. Rheumatol.* **2012**, *41*, 150–155. [CrossRef] [PubMed]
6. Martinez-Calderon, J.; Struyf, F.; Meeus, M.; Morales-Ascencio, J.M.; Luque-Suarez, A. Influence of psychological factors on the prognosis of chronic shoulder pain: Protocol for a prospective cohort study. *BMJ Open* **2017**, *7*, e012822. [CrossRef] [PubMed]
7. Yang, S.; Kim, T.U.; Kim, D.H.; Chang, M.C. Understanding the physical examination of the shoulder: A narrative review. *Ann. Palliat. Med.* **2021**, *10*, 2293–2303. [CrossRef] [PubMed]
8. Osborne, J.D.; Gowda, A.L.; Wiater, B.; Wiater, J.M. Rotator cuff rehabilitation: Current theories and practice. *Phys. Sportsmed.* **2016**, *44*, 85–92. [CrossRef]
9. Garving, C.; Jakob, S.; Bauer, I.; Nadjar, R.; Brunner, U.H. Impingement Syndrome of the Shoulder. *Dtsch. Arztebl. Int.* **2017**, *114*, 765–776. [CrossRef]
10. Greenberg, D.L. Evaluation and treatment of shoulder pain. *Med. Clin. N. Am.* **2014**, *98*, 487–504. [CrossRef]
11. Garibaldi, R.; Altomare, D.; Sconza, C.; Kon, E.; Castagna, A.; Marcacci, M.; Monina, E.; Di Matteo, B. Conservative management vs. surgical repair in degenerative rotator cuff tears: A systematic review and meta-analysis. *Eur. Rev. Med. Pharmacol. Sci.* **2021**, *25*, 609–619. [CrossRef] [PubMed]
12. Kuijpers, T.; van der Windt, D.; van der Heijden, G.; Bouter, L.M. Systematic review of prognostic cohort studies on shoulder disorders. *Pain* **2004**, *109*, 420–431. [CrossRef] [PubMed]
13. Boersma, K.; Linton, S.J. Expectancy, fear and pain in the prediction of chronic pain and disability: A prospective analysis. *Eur. J. Pain* **2006**, *10*, 551–557. [CrossRef] [PubMed]
14. Luque-Suarez, A.; Martinez-Calderon, J.; Navarro-Ledesma, S.; Morales-Asencio, J.M.; Meeus, M.; Struyf, F. Kinesiophobia Is Associated With Pain Intensity and Disability in Chronic Shoulder Pain: A Cross-Sectional Study. *J. Manip. Physiol. Ther.* **2020**, *43*, 791–798. [CrossRef] [PubMed]
15. Thorpe, A.M.; O'Sullivan, P.B.; Mitchell, T.; Hurworth, M.; Spencer, J.; Booth, G.; Goebel, S.; Khoo, P.; Tay, A.; Smith, A. Are Psychologic Factors Associated With Shoulder Scores After Rotator Cuff Surgery? *Clin. Orthop. Relat. Res.* **2018**, *476*, 2062–2073. [CrossRef] [PubMed]
16. Meulders, A.; Vlaeyen, J.W.S. The acquisition and generalization of cued and contextual pain-related fear: An experimental study using a voluntary movement paradigm. *Pain* **2013**, *154*, 272–282. [CrossRef] [PubMed]
17. Vlaeyen, J.W.S. Learning to predict and control harmful events: Chronic pain and conditioning. *Pain* **2015**, *156* (Suppl. S1), S86–S93. [CrossRef] [PubMed]
18. Bordeleau, M.; Vincenot, M.; Lefevre, S.; Duport, A.; Seggio, L.; Breton, T.; Lelard, T.; Serra, E.; Roussel, N.; Neves, J.F.D.; et al. Treatments for kinesiophobia in people with chronic pain: A scoping review. *Front. Behav. Neurosci.* **2022**, *16*, 933483. [CrossRef] [PubMed]

19. Cuff, A.; Littlewood, C. Subacromial impingement syndrome—What does this mean to and for the patient? A qualitative study. *Musculoskelet. Sci. Pract.* **2018**, *33*, 24–28. [CrossRef]
20. Miller, J.E.; Higgins, L.D.; Dong, Y.; Collins, J.E.; Bean, J.F.; Seitz, A.L.; Katz, J.N.; Jain, N.B. Association of Strength Measurement with Rotator Cuff Tear in Patients with Shoulder Pain: The Rotator Cuff Outcomes Workgroup Study. *Am. J. Phys. Med. Rehabil.* **2016**, *95*, 47–56. [CrossRef]
21. Miller, J.; MacDermid, J.C.; Richardson, J.; Walton, D.M.; Gross, A. Depicting individual responses to physical therapist led chronic pain self-management support with pain science education and exercise in primary health care: Multiple case studies. *Arch. Physiother.* **2017**, *7*, 4. [CrossRef]
22. Briggs, E. Evaluating the impact of pain education: How do we know we have made a difference? *Br. J. Pain* **2012**, *6*, 85–91. [CrossRef]
23. Lepri, B.; Romani, D.; Storari, L.; Barbari, V. Effectiveness of Pain Neuroscience Education in Patients with Chronic Musculoskeletal Pain and Central Sensitization: A Systematic Review. *Int. J. Environ. Res. Public Health* **2023**, *20*, 4098. [CrossRef] [PubMed]
24. Nijs, J.; Paul van Wilgen, C.; Van Oosterwijck, J.; van Ittersum, M.; Meeus, M. How to explain central sensitization to patients with 'unexplained' chronic musculoskeletal pain: Practice guidelines. *Man. Ther.* **2011**, *16*, 413–418. [CrossRef] [PubMed]
25. Watson, J.A.; Ryan, C.G.; Cooper, L.; Ellington, D.; Whittle, R.; Lavender, M.; Dixon, J.; Atkinson, G.; Cooper, K.; Martin, D.J. Pain Neuroscience Education for Adults With Chronic Musculoskeletal Pain: A Mixed-Methods Systematic Review and Meta-Analysis. *J. Pain.* **2019**, *20*, 1140.e11–1140.e22. [CrossRef] [PubMed]
26. Varallo, G.; Suso-Ribera, C.; Ghiggia, A.; Veneruso, M.; Cattivelli, R.; Guerrini Usubini, A.; Franceschini, C.; Musetti, A.; Plazzi, G.; Fontana, J.M.; et al. Catastrophizing, Kinesiophobia, and Acceptance as Mediators of the Relationship Between Perceived Pain Severity, Self-Reported and Performance-Based Physical Function in Women with Fibromyalgia and Obesity. *J. Pain Res.* **2022**, *15*, 3017–3029. [CrossRef] [PubMed]
27. Galan-Martin, M.A.; Montero-Cuadrado, F.; Lluch-Girbes, E.; Coca-Lopez, M.C.; Mayo-Iscar, A.; Cuesta-Vargas, A. Pain Neuroscience Education and Physical Therapeutic Exercise for Patients with Chronic Spinal Pain in Spanish Physiotherapy Primary Care: A Pragmatic Randomized Controlled Trial. *J. Clin. Med.* **2020**, *9*, 1201. [CrossRef] [PubMed]
28. Diener, I.; Kargela, M.; Louw, A. Listening is therapy: Patient interviewing from a pain science perspective. *Physiother. Theory Pract.* **2016**, *32*, 356–367. [CrossRef]
29. Alito, A.; Verme, F.; Mercati, G.P.; Piterà, P.; Fontana, J.M.; Capodaglio, P. Whole Body Cryostimulation: A New Adjuvant Treatment in Central Sensitization Syndromes? An Expert Opinion. *Healthcare* **2024**, *12*, 546. [CrossRef]
30. Fontana, J.M.; Alito, A.; Piterà, P.; Verme, F.; Cattaldo, S.; Cornacchia, M.; Mai, S.; Brunani, A.; Capodaglio, P. Whole-Body Cryostimulation in Post-COVID Rehabilitation for Patients with Obesity: A Multidisciplinary Feasibility Study. *Biomedicines* **2023**, *11*, 3092. [CrossRef]
31. Varallo, G.; Piterà, P.; Fontana, J.M.; Gobbi, M.; Arreghini, M.; Giusti, E.M.; Franceschini, C.; Plazzi, G.; Castelnuovo, G.; Capodaglio, P. Is Whole-Body Cryostimulation an Effective Add-On Treatment in Individuals with Fibromyalgia and Obesity? A Randomized Controlled Clinical Trial. *J. Clin. Med.* **2022**, *11*, 4324. [CrossRef] [PubMed]
32. Piterà, P.; Springhetti, I.; Alito, A.; Verme, F.; Fontana, J.M.; Capodaglio, P. Whole-Body Cryostimulation, a Complementary Treatment for Phantom Limb Syndrome: Preliminary Evidence from a Case Study. *Medicina* **2024**, *60*, 22. [CrossRef] [PubMed]
33. Bouzigon, R.; Dupuy, O.; Tiemessen, I.; De Nardi, M.; Bernard, J.P.; Mihailovic, T.; Theurot, D.; Miller, E.D.; Lombardi, G.; Dugué, B.M. Cryostimulation for Post-exercise Recovery in Athletes: A Consensus and Position Paper. *Front. Sports Act. Living* **2021**, *3*, 688828. [CrossRef] [PubMed]
34. Riley, D.S.; Barber, M.S.; Kienle, G.S.; Aronson, J.K.; von Schoen-Angerer, T.; Tugwell, P.; Kiene, H.; Helfand, M.; Altman, D.G.; Sox, H.; et al. CARE guidelines for case reports: Explanation and elaboration document. *J. Clin. Epidemiol.* **2017**, *89*, 218–235. [CrossRef] [PubMed]
35. Enright, P.L. The six-minute walk test. *Respir. Care* **2003**, *48*, 783–785.
36. Amaral, C.A.; Amaral, T.L.M.; Monteiro, G.T.R.; Vasconcellos, M.T.L.; Portela, M.C. Hand grip strength: Reference values for adults and elderly people of Rio Branco, Acre, Brazil. *PLoS ONE* **2019**, *14*, e0211452. [CrossRef] [PubMed]
37. Grossi, E.; Compare, A. Psychological General Well-Being Index (PGWB). In *Encyclopedia of Quality of Life and Well-Being Research*; Michalos, A.C., Ed.; Springer: Dordrecht, The Netherlands, 2014; pp. 5152–5156.
38. Gummesson, C.; Atroshi, I.; Ekdahl, C. The disabilities of the arm, shoulder and hand (DASH) outcome questionnaire: Longitudinal construct validity and measuring self-rated health change after surgery. *BMC Musculoskelet. Disord.* **2003**, *4*, 11. [CrossRef]
39. Breckenridge, J.D.; McAuley, J.H. Shoulder Pain and Disability Index (SPADI). *J. Physiother.* **2011**, *57*, 197. [CrossRef]
40. Ware, J.E., Jr. SF-36 Health Survey. In *The Use of Psychological Testing for Treatment Planning and Outcomes Assessment*, 2nd ed.; Lawrence Erlbaum Associates Publishers: Mahwah, NJ, USA, 1999; pp. 1227–1246.
41. Hudes, K. The Tampa Scale of Kinesiophobia and neck pain, disability and range of motion: A narrative review of the literature. *J. Can. Chiropr. Assoc.* **2011**, *55*, 222–232.
42. Mills, S.E.E.; Nicolson, K.P.; Smith, B.H. Chronic pain: A review of its epidemiology and associated factors in population-based studies. *Br. J. Anaesth.* **2019**, *123*, e273–e283. [CrossRef]
43. Asmundson, G.J.G.; Parkerson, H.A.; D'Ambrosio, C.A. Fear, Anxiety, Avoidance, and Chronic Pain. In *Anxiety Disorders*; Ressler, K.J., Pine, D.S., Rothbaum, B.O., Eds.; Oxford University Press: Oxford, UK, 2015; pp. 227–240.

44. Li, L.; Sun, Y.; Qin, H.; Zhou, J.; Yang, X.; Li, A.; Zhang, J.; Zhang, Y. A scientometric analysis and visualization of kinesiophobia research from 2002 to 2022: A review. *Medicine* **2023**, *102*, e35872. [CrossRef] [PubMed]
45. Bränström, H.; Fahlström, M. Kinesiophobia in patients with chronic musculoskeletal pain: Differences between men and women. *J. Rehabil. Med.* **2008**, *40*, 375–380. [CrossRef] [PubMed]
46. Luque-Suarez, A.; Martinez-Calderon, J.; Falla, D. Role of kinesiophobia on pain, disability and quality of life in people suffering from chronic musculoskeletal pain: A systematic review. *Br. J. Sports Med.* **2019**, *53*, 554–559. [CrossRef] [PubMed]
47. Wang, Q.; Du, N. Relationship between kinesiophobia and quality of life among patients with breast cancer–related lymphedema: Chain-mediating effect of self-care and functional exercise compliance. *Asia-Pac. J. Oncol. Nurs.* **2024**, *11*, 100346. [CrossRef] [PubMed]
48. White, G.E.; Wells, G.D. Cold-water immersion and other forms of cryotherapy: Physiological changes potentially affecting recovery from high-intensity exercise. *Extrem. Physiol. Med.* **2013**, *2*, 26. [CrossRef] [PubMed]
49. Banfi, G.; Melegati, G.; Barassi, A.; Dogliotti, G.; d'Eril, G.M.; Dugué, B.; Corsi, M.M. Effects of whole-body cryotherapy on serum mediators of inflammation and serum muscle enzymes in athletes. *J. Therm. Biol.* **2009**, *34*, 55–59. [CrossRef]
50. Ma, S.Y.; Je, H.D.; Jeong, J.H.; Kim, H.Y.; Kim, H.D. Effects of whole-body cryotherapy in the management of adhesive capsulitis of the shoulder. *Arch. Phys. Med. Rehabil.* **2013**, *94*, 9–16. [CrossRef] [PubMed]
51. Alito, A.; Quartarone, A.; Leonardi, G.; Tisano, A.; Bruschetta, A.; Cucinotta, F.; Milardi, D.; Portaro, S. Brown adipose tissue human biomarkers: Which one fits best? A narrative review. *Medicine* **2022**, *101*, e32181. [CrossRef]
52. Douzi, W.; Dupuy, O.; Theurot, D.; Boucard, G.; Dugué, B. Partial-body cryostimulation after training improves sleep quality in professional soccer players. *BMC Res. Notes* **2019**, *12*, 141. [CrossRef]
53. Louis, J.; Theurot, D.; Filliard, J.-R.; Volondat, M.; Dugué, B.; Dupuy, O. The use of whole-body cryotherapy: Time- and dose-response investigation on circulating blood catecholamines and heart rate variability. *Eur. J. Appl. Physiol.* **2020**, *120*, 1733–1743. [CrossRef]
54. Verme, F.; Fontana, J.M.; Piterà, P.; Alito, A.; Saffioti, S.; Baccalaro, G.; Zebellin, G.; Capodaglio, P. Whole-Body Cryostimulation in Functional Neurological Disorders: A Case Report. *Healthcare* **2023**, *12*, 71. [CrossRef] [PubMed]
55. Larsson, C.; Ekvall Hansson, E.; Sundquist, K.; Jakobsson, U. Kinesiophobia and its relation to pain characteristics and cognitive affective variables in older adults with chronic pain. *BMC Geriatr.* **2016**, *16*, 128. [CrossRef] [PubMed]
56. Heuts, P.H.; Vlaeyen, J.W.; Roelofs, J.; de Bie, R.A.; Aretz, K.; van Weel, C.; van Schayck, O.C. Pain-related fear and daily functioning in patients with osteoarthritis. *Pain* **2004**, *110*, 228–235. [CrossRef] [PubMed]
57. Suso-Martí, L.; Cuenca-Martínez, F.; Alba-Quesada, P.; Muñoz-Alarcos, V.; Herranz-Gómez, A.; Varangot-Reille, C.; Domínguez-Navarro, F.; Casaña, J. Effectiveness of Pain Neuroscience Education in Patients with Fibromyalgia: A Systematic Review and Meta-Analysis. *Pain Med.* **2022**, *23*, 1837–1850. [CrossRef] [PubMed]

Journal of
Clinical Medicine

MDPI

Article

AI in Hand Surgery: Assessing Large Language Models in the Classification and Management of Hand Injuries

Sophia M. Pressman [1], Sahar Borna [1], Cesar A. Gomez-Cabello [1], Syed Ali Haider [1] and Antonio Jorge Forte [1,2,*]

[1] Division of Plastic Surgery, Mayo Clinic, Jacksonville, FL 32224, USA; sophiampressman1@gmail.com (S.M.P.); saharborna2021@gmail.com (S.B.); abrahamgomezcabello@gmail.com (C.A.G.-C.); dr.s.alihaider@gmail.com (S.A.H.)
[2] Center for Digital Health, Mayo Clinic, Rochester, MN 55905, USA
* Correspondence: ajvforte@yahoo.com.br

Abstract: Background: OpenAI's ChatGPT (San Francisco, CA, USA) and Google's Gemini (Mountain View, CA, USA) are two large language models that show promise in improving and expediting medical decision making in hand surgery. Evaluating the applications of these models within the field of hand surgery is warranted. This study aims to evaluate ChatGPT-4 and Gemini in classifying hand injuries and recommending treatment. **Methods**: Gemini and ChatGPT were given 68 fictionalized clinical vignettes of hand injuries twice. The models were asked to use a specific classification system and recommend surgical or nonsurgical treatment. Classifications were scored based on correctness. Results were analyzed using descriptive statistics, a paired two-tailed *t*-test, and sensitivity testing. **Results**: Gemini, correctly classifying 70.6% hand injuries, demonstrated superior classification ability over ChatGPT (mean score 1.46 vs. 0.87, p-value < 0.001). For management, ChatGPT demonstrated higher sensitivity in recommending surgical intervention compared to Gemini (98.0% vs. 88.8%), but lower specificity (68.4% vs. 94.7%). When compared to ChatGPT, Gemini demonstrated greater response replicability. **Conclusions**: Large language models like ChatGPT and Gemini show promise in assisting medical decision making, particularly in hand surgery, with Gemini generally outperforming ChatGPT. These findings emphasize the importance of considering the strengths and limitations of different models when integrating them into clinical practice.

Keywords: artificial intelligence (AI); ChatGPT; Gemini; deep learning; machine learning; hand surgery; hand trauma; management

1. Introduction

The integration of artificial intelligence (AI) into daily medical practice is an evitable reality [1,2]. With an expanding repertoire of applications and tools, AI is infiltrating the healthcare landscape, seeping into every specialty and healthcare domain [3,4]. This progression is marked by the emergence of large language models (LLMs). Built upon neural network architectures [5], LLMs are AI systems which are designed to employ deep learning and natural language processing [6]. These models undergo extensive training on vast datasets until they are able to comprehend and generate human-like text with significant predictability [6], even without employing retrieval-augmented generation (RAG) approaches. Two publicly available LLMs that have garnered recent interest are Google's Gemini [7] (built upon its predecessor Bard) and OpenAI's ChatGPT [8]. Although not designed specifically for medical purposes, these LLMs have demonstrated potential in medical decision making [9]. For example, ChatGPT achieved passing scores for both the United States Medical Licensing Examination [10] and American Society for Surgery of the Hand self-assessment exam [11], demonstrating a basic level of competence in medical reasoning. With the potential to enhance diagnostic accuracy, informed decision making, and patient outcomes, LLMs like ChatGPT and Gemini show promise in augmenting healthcare delivery [9,12].

The field of hand surgery stands to benefit greatly from the support of AI tools like LLMs [1,13]. Achieving favorable outcomes after hand trauma is paramount, given the critical role that hands play in necessary tasks for daily functioning and independence [14–17]. Effective management relies heavily on correctly identifying the nature and severity of injuries, as this information guides decisions regarding surgical intervention, rehabilitation, and ongoing care [18–21]. Inaccurate diagnosis and classification can lead to delays in treatment, inappropriate interventions, and potentially compromised functional recovery for patients [22,23]. With their advanced algorithms, LLMs can analyze complex patterns [6] and thus have the potential to provide rapid and precise injury classifications, enhancing and expediting the management process.

While the integration of advanced LLMs into healthcare systems is on the horizon, access may be limited to those within those institutions. Healthcare professionals in underfunded facilities, medical students, and patients are expected to continue using publicly available LLMs like ChatGPT and Gemini for medical queries. The continuous assessment of the value and utility of these LLMs is essential. Early investigations into LLM applications in hand surgery have shown promising results. Leypold et al. [24] found that ChatGPT adeptly managed complex hand and arm surgery scenarios, showcasing the potential of LLMs like ChatGPT to improve patient care and surgical outcomes. Crook et al. [25] reported ChatGPT's proficiency in addressing common patient inquiries regarding common hand surgeries, noting generally high-quality responses. In a similar study, Seth et al. [26] found that ChatGPT was suitable for nonmedical individuals, but struggled with accurate and complete references. Additionally, Al Rawi et al. [27] observed that, while ChatGPT's responses were correct and useful in most cases, only 57% were deemed complete by hand surgeon reviewers.

Although these studies show promise for ChatGPT, there is limited research exploring Gemini's potential in hand surgery and few studies comparing LLMs. Furthermore, additional research to explore the full extent of LLM capabilities in the context of hand injuries and hand surgery, particularly in specialized tasks like injury classification, is warranted. The objective of this study is to assess the ability of ChatGPT and Gemini to accurately classify hand injuries via the use of 12 specific classification systems. Furthermore, this study aims to determine the ability of these models to accurately recommend surgical or nonsurgical management for these hand injuries. In doing so, we seek to evaluate the capabilities of publicly available LLMs without the use of RAG approaches. Through this investigation, this study endeavors to advance the ongoing discourse surrounding the applications and limitations of LLMs in hand surgery.

2. Materials and Methods

2.1. Study Design

Sixty-eight unique prompts were developed to test each LLM's ability to classify hand injuries. Prompts cover 12 different classification systems [20,21,28–39] covering various hand injuries. The inclusion criteria prioritized classification systems with well-established significance, ensuring relevance and familiarity among healthcare providers specializing in hand surgery. To focus on clinically relevant systems, classification systems lacking direct treatment correlations were excluded.

Each prompt was prefaced with, "I am a plastic and reconstructive surgeon who specializes in hand surgery. You are my colleague and I am discussing a case with you." Each prompt included a fictionalized vignette and a specific hand injury diagnosis. Additionally, within each prompt was a request to classify the injury using a specific classification system and determine if this injury warrants surgical or nonsurgical (conservative) management. The deliberate inclusion of the specific diagnosis and classification system of interest was incorporated to focus the evaluation of the LLMs' classification abilities, rather than their diagnostic skills, ensuring a uniform methodology and reducing the likelihood of LLMs using varying classification systems. Examples of prompts with LLM responses are depicted in Figures 1 and 2. Each prompt was provided to ChatGPT-4 (OpenAI, San Francisco, CA, USA) and Gemini (Google, Mountain View, CA, USA) twice to ensure consistency and replicability, resulting in a total of 136 prompts. Additionally, each prompt was entered individually in a separate conversation to minimize the possibility of one answer affecting another. All prompts were provided on 10 March 2024, using the Google Chrome internet browser.

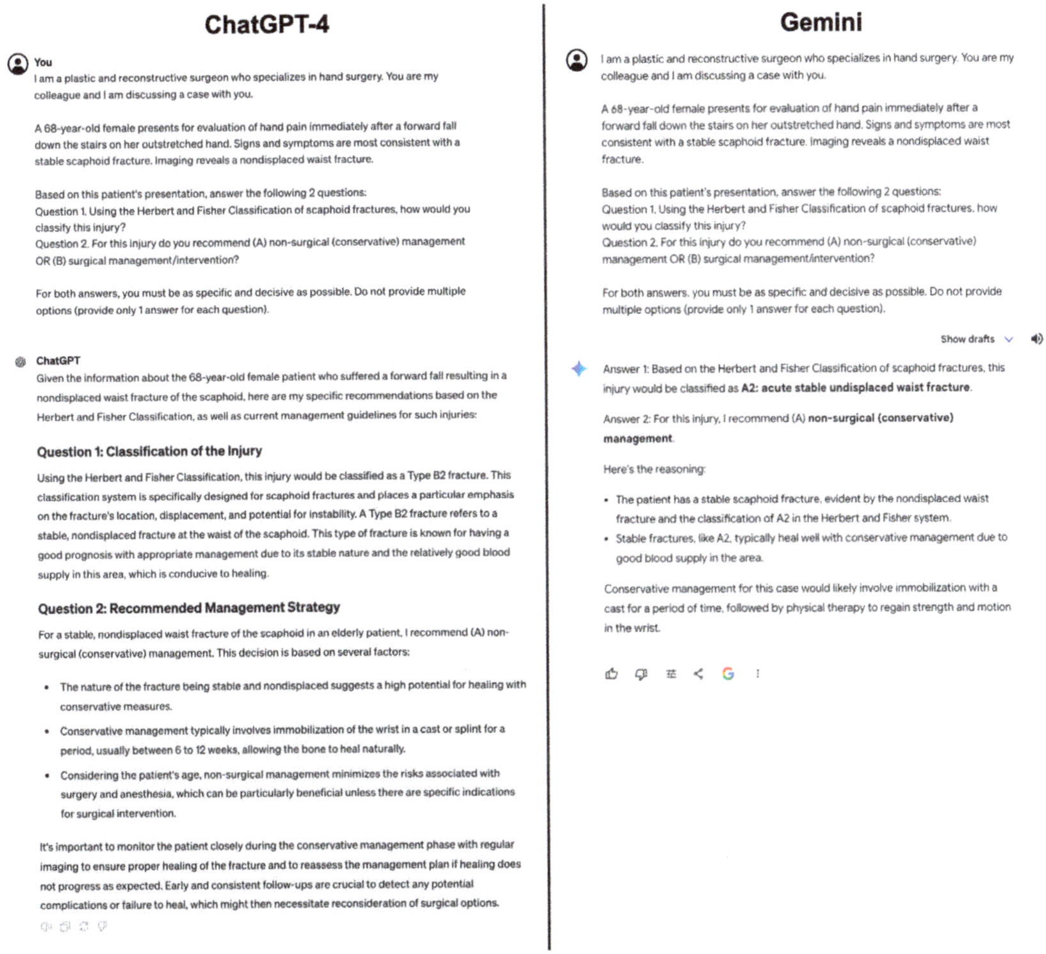

Figure 1. An example of a prompt given to ChatGPT-4 (**left**) and Gemini (**right**) with the corresponding responses below. This prompt asked the models to classify a scaphoid fracture using Herbert and Fisher's classification system.

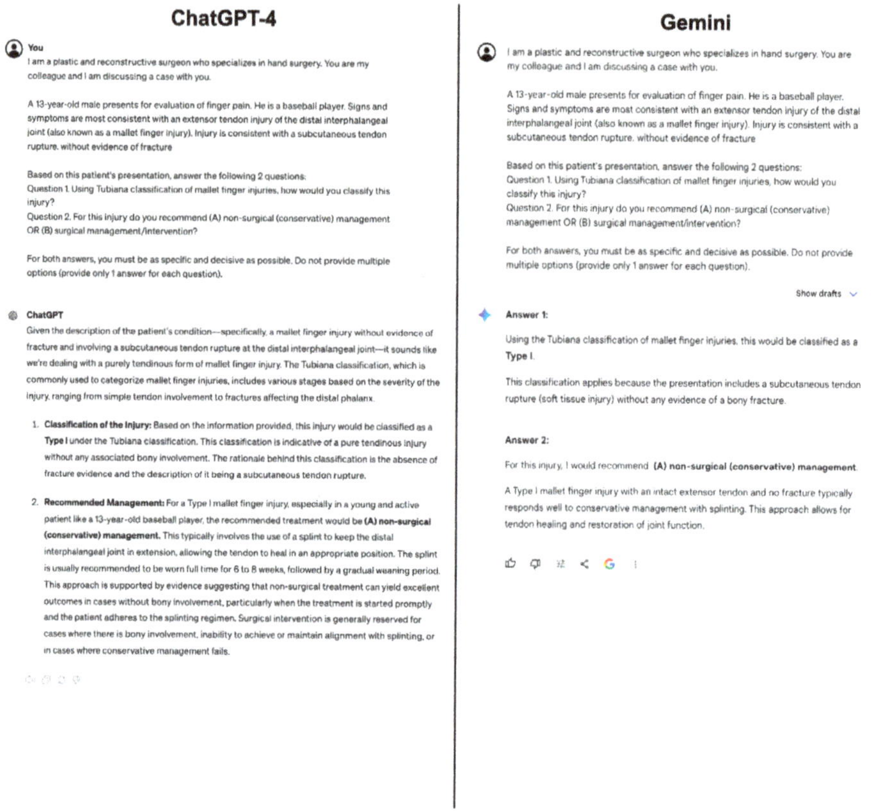

Figure 2. An example of a prompt given to ChatGPT-4 (**left**) and Gemini (**right**) with the corresponding responses. This prompt asked the models to classify a mallet finger injury using Tubiana's classification system.

For the assessment of classification abilities, the LLMs were given points based on answer correctness. Completely correct classifications were awarded two points, partially correct classifications were awarded one point, and incorrect classifications were awarded zero points. Instances of partial correctness typically arose from either indecisiveness on the part of the LLM or from including subclassifications within the classification system. For example, in systems like the Gustilo–Anderson classification [20,33] for open fractures, which have subclassifications (e.g., Type IIIA, IIIB, and IIIC), partial correctness could result from selecting the wrong subclassification (e.g., selecting Type IIIB when the correct answer was Type IIIA) or from failing to specify the subclassification altogether (e.g., answering Type III when the correct answer was Type IIIA). Furthermore, if the LLM struggled to choose between two options, one of which was correct, it would still receive one point for partial correctness.

In our investigation into the LLM's ability to differentiate between surgical and nonsurgical management options for hand injuries, we relied on clinically pertinent classification systems as our gold standard. These classification systems were chosen for their comprehensive treatment recommendations which were associated with each categorized injury. As such, the recommendations provided within the classification systems served as the definitive 'correct' answers for our study. Furthermore, to ensure the accuracy of our assessments, all responses were verified by a board-certified hand surgeon. By adhering to these established guidelines, we aimed to maintain consistency and objectivity in our evaluation process. This approach not only provided a clear framework for comparing LLM performance, but also ensured the clinical relevance and validity of our findings.

2.2. Data Collection and Analysis

Prompts and corresponding LLM responses were collected in Microsoft Excel (Redmond, WA, USA). Each response was graded based on classification correctness. These values were analyzed using descriptive statistics including the mean, standard deviation (SD), and range. Comparisons between ChatGPT and Gemini classification abilities were evaluated using paired, two-tailed *t*-tests. This test controls for variability across different clinical vignettes and allows for the detection of significant differences, without assuming directionality. Subgroup analyses were conducted to compare scores for each classification system. An alpha level of 0.05 was used to determine statistical significance.

In addition to classification accuracy, the evaluation of the LLMs' capacity to recommend surgical versus nonsurgical management involved the calculation of sensitivity (also known as recall), specificity, positive predictive value (PPV; also known as precision), accuracy, and the F1 score. Sensitivity and specificity offer insights into the models' ability to accurately identify true surgical and nonsurgical cases, respectively, while PPV and accuracy shed light on the precision and correctness of the models' recommendations. Furthermore, the F1 score serves as a synthesized measure, capturing the balance between precision and recall, and offering a more nuanced understanding of the models' overall performance. This multifaceted evaluation approach ensures that the strengths and weaknesses of the LLMs' recommendations are thoroughly explored, providing valuable insights for healthcare providers and researchers alike in navigating the complexities of decision making in hand surgery.

3. Results

3.1. Classification Results

In the classification of hand injuries, Gemini exhibited superior performance over ChatGPT, with an average score of 1.46 (SD 0.87), whereas ChatGPT yielded an average score of 0.67 (SD 0.87) (p-value < 0.001). Classification results are displayed in Table 1 and Figure 3. Gemini provided completely correct classifications for 96 (70.6%) hand injuries, but partially correct and incorrect for six (4.4%) and 34 (25.0%) injuries, respectively. ChatGPT provided correct, partially correct, and incorrect classifications for 36 (26.5%), 19 (14.0%), and 81 (59.6%) hand injuries, respectively.

ChatGPT exhibited its strongest performance in utilizing the Lichtman classification [38] for Kienböck disease (osteonecrosis of the lunate), correctly classifying eight cases (66.7%) with a mean score of 1.58 (SD 0.67). Additionally, its next best performance was in employing the Gustilo–Anderson classification [20,33] for open fractures, accurately categorizing seven cases (70%) with a mean score of 1.50 (SD 0.85). However, its performance was notably poorer when using Hintermann et al.'s classification [35] system for Gamekeeper's thumb, where all of its classifications were incorrect. Similarly, ChatGPT struggled with the classification of scaphoid fractures, where it inaccurately classified all cases according to the Mayo classification [28,29] system. Furthermore, in classifying volar plate avulsion injuries using the Eaton classification [30] system, ChatGPT demonstrated unacceptable performance, failing to correctly classify any cases. In contrast, Gemini displayed superior classification capabilities, providing accurate classifications for all volar plate avulsion injuries using the Eaton classification [30] system and all scaphoid fractures using the Herbert and Fisher Classification [34]. Despite this, Gemini's weakest performance was observed when classifying flexor tendon injuries using Kleinert and Verdan's Zone classification [36] system. Notably, ChatGPT narrowly outperformed Gemini only in the Gustilo–Anderson classification [20,33] of open fractures, Kleinert and Verdan's Zone classification [36] of flexor tendon injuries, and the Lichtman classification [38] for Kienböck disease (osteonecrosis of the lunate).

Table 1. Hand injury classification results from the LLMs.

Classification System	LLM	Correct	Partially Correct	Incorrect	Mean Score	Standard Deviation
Eaton classification for volar plate avulsion injuries	ChatGPT-4 Gemini	0 8	1 0	7 0	0.13 2.00	0.35 0.00
Geissler arthroscopic classification for carpal instability	ChatGPT-4 Gemini	3 4	0 0	5 4	0.75 1.00	1.04 1.07
Green and O'Brien's classification of thumb metacarpal fractures	ChatGPT-4 Gemini	1 11	1 1	10 0	0.25 1.92	0.62 0.29
Gustilo-Anderson classification of open fractures	ChatGPT-4 Gemini	7 5	1 3	2 2	1.50 1.30	0.85 0.82
Herbert and Fisher Classification of scaphoid fractures	ChatGPT-4 Gemini	4 20	6 0	10 0	0.70 2.00	0.80 0.00
Hintermann et al.'s classification of ulnar collateral ligament (UCL) injury of the thumb	ChatGPT-4 Gemini	0 10	0 0	12 2	0.00 1.67	0.00 0.78
Kleinert and Verdan's Zone classification of flexor tendon injuries	ChatGPT-4 Gemini	3 4	6 2	7 10	0.75 0.63	0.77 0.89
Leddy and Packer classification of avulsion injury of the flexor digitorum profundus (FDP)	ChatGPT-4 Gemini	4 6	0 0	8 6	0.67 1.00	0.98 1.04
Lichtman classification of Kienböck disease (osteonecrosis the lunate)	ChatGPT-4 Gemini	8 8	3 0	1 4	1.58 1.33	0.67 0.98
Mayfield classification for carpal instability	ChatGPT-4 Gemini	4 6	1 0	3 2	1.13 1.50	0.99 0.93
Mayo Classification of scaphoid fractures	ChatGPT-4 Gemini	0 8	0 0	10 2	0.00 1.60	0.00 0.84
Tubiana classification for mallet finger	ChatGPT-4 Gemini	2 6	0 0	6 2	0.50 1.50	0.93 0.93
Total	ChatGPT-4 Gemini	36 96	19 6	81 34	0.67 1.46	0.87 0.87

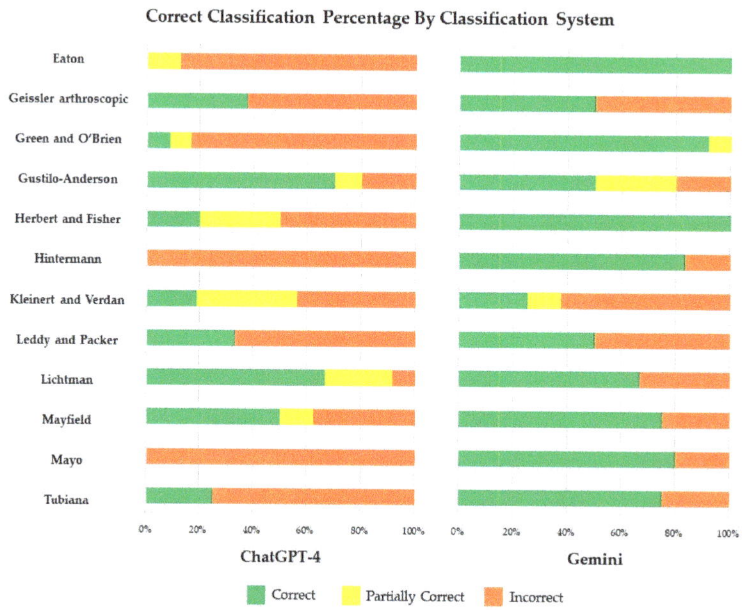

Figure 3. Percentage of correct classifications for each classification system for ChatGPT-4 (**left**) and Gemini (**right**).

3.2. Surgical Management Results from Sensitivity Testing

Based on the clinical vignettes and classification, 98 (72.1%) injuries warranted surgical intervention, and 38 (27.9%) justified nonsurgical management. ChatGPT recommended surgical intervention for 108 (79.4%) cases, as compared to Gemini, which recommended surgery for only 89 (65.4%). The results of the sensitivity testing are shown in Table 2. ChatGPT demonstrated higher sensitivity (recall) in recommending surgical intervention when compared to Gemini (98.0% vs. 88.8%). However, Gemini demonstrated a specificity of 94.7%, which was higher than ChatGPT's specificity of 68.4%. Additionally, Gemini demonstrated a PPV (precision) of 97.8%, which was higher than ChatGPT's PPV of 88.9%. Both models exhibited comparable F1 scores, with ChatGPT achieving an F1 score of 0.932 and Gemini achieving an F1 score of 0.930.

Table 2. Results of sensitivity testing.

Value	ChatGPT	Gemini
Sensitivity	0.980	0.888
Specificity	0.684	0.947
Positive Predictive Value (PPV)	0.889	0.978
Negative Predictive Value (NPV)	0.929	0.766
Positive Likelihood Ratio (LR+)	3.102	16.867
Negative Likelihood Ratio (LR−)	0.030	0.118
Accuracy	0.897	0.904
F1 score	0.932	0.930

3.3. Replicability Results

To ensure consistency, each of the 68 prompts was presented twice. Gemini's classification response differed in six instances (8.9%). In contrast, ChatGPT showed more variability, with its classification changing in 17 cases (25.0%), indicating a lower level of consistency and replicability. Among ChatGPT's changes, 12 (70.5%) resulted in a more accurate classification (e.g., changing from incorrect to partially correct, changing from incorrect to correct, or changing from partially correct to correct). In terms of recommending surgical or nonsurgical management, ChatGPT modified its answer for six (8.9%) injuries, five of which were corrected in the subsequent response. However, Gemini's response changed only once (1.5%), albeit to the incorrect management choice.

4. Discussion

With the correct classification of 70.6% of hand injuries, Gemini demonstrated superior performance to ChatGPT, which correctly classified just over a quarter of the injuries. ChatGPT's poor performance, specifically when using the Eaton [30], Hintermann [35], and Mayo [28,29] classification systems, may suggest a lack of information relating to these classification systems in the dataset on which it was trained. The results of this study demonstrate Gemini's superior performance over ChatGPT, which contrasts the few prior comparative studies involving Gemini, where ChatGPT was found to demonstrate greater accuracy [40,41]. Similarly, previous studies comparing ChatGPT to Gemini's predecessor, Bard, have shown varied results, with some studies favoring ChatGPT [42–45] and others favoring Bard [46,47]. Without a definitive accuracy threshold, neither model is currently reliable enough as a classification tool to be used in clinical practice, but this situation is expected to change shortly. While neither ChatGPT nor Gemini were designed for medical use, the findings reveal promising potential in hand injury classification, which is just one of its potential applications in hand surgery (Figure 4). With the further expansion of datasets and the refinement of algorithms, these models are anticipated to reach the required level of accuracy for practical use.

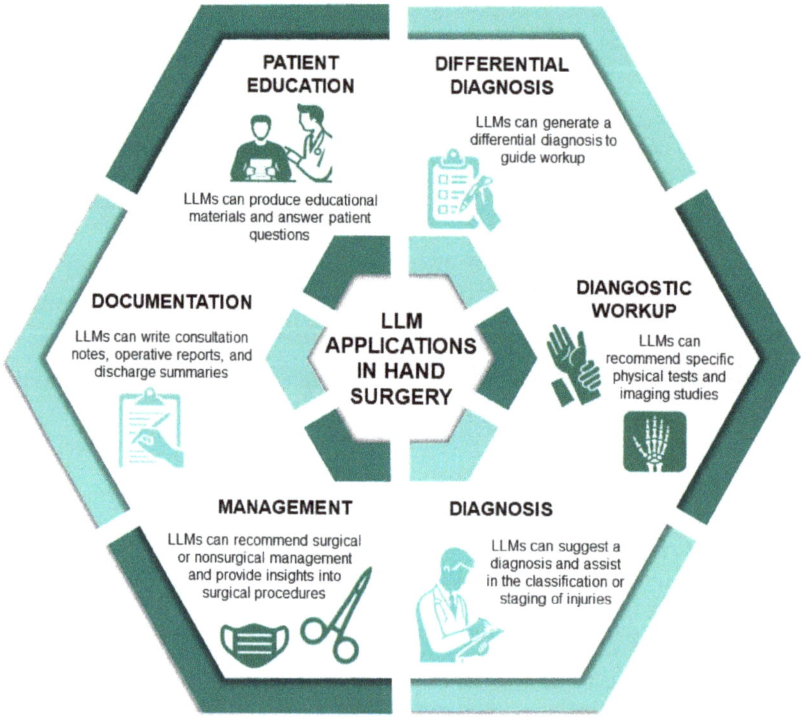

Figure 4. Applications of large language models (LLMs) in hand surgery.

The findings from sensitivity testing indicate that ChatGPT leans towards recommending surgical intervention more quickly, whereas Gemini takes a more cautious and conservative approach, showing hesitation in recommending surgical intervention. These differing behaviors carry significant implications, particularly in clinical decision-making scenarios. While ChatGPT's promptness may offer a sense of urgency, it also raises concerns regarding the potential for the over-recommendation of surgical procedures. On the other hand, Gemini's reluctance may contribute to a more conservative approach, minimizing the risk of unnecessary interventions, but possibly at the expense of timely action when surgical intervention is indeed warranted. Healthcare providers must carefully consider these nuances when incorporating AI decision-support tools into clinical practice, balancing the need for prompt action with the importance of exercising prudence and minimizing unnecessary interventions.

When compared to ChatGPT, Gemini also demonstrated greater consistency in its answers. This is not unsurprising, as previous studies [48–50] have reported concerns regarding ChatGPT's consistency. To be a reliable medical resource, an LLM must ensure that its prompts and recommendations are reproducible, replicable, and consistent across diverse interactions and contexts. Achieving this ensures that healthcare providers can trust the model's outputs consistently, thereby streamlining their decision-making processes [50]. This enhanced reliability not only instills confidence in the LLM's capabilities, but also translates into more efficient and effective patient care, as clinicians can rely on the model to provide accurate and consistent guidance in various medical scenarios.

Although not the main focus of this study, it was evident that ChatGPT tended to generate lengthy and verbose responses, whereas Gemini provided more concise ones. In a clinical environment, where healthcare providers are frequently pressed for time and efficiency is paramount, the ability to deliver concise responses can be highly beneficial.

Given that every minute counts in such settings, the succinctness of Gemini's responses may offer a practical advantage, enabling healthcare professionals to quickly grasp essential information without unnecessary verbosity. In the high-pressure setting of the emergency department (ED), where healthcare providers are often inundated with urgent cases, the rapid delivery of concise, accurate information would be especially beneficial. Gemini's capability to provide succinct responses can support emergency providers in quickly assessing and prioritizing cases, thus enabling efficient resource allocation and expediting critical interventions.

ED applications of LLMs thus far have mostly focused on evaluating ChatGPT's ability to triage and diagnose. Berg et al. [48] examined ChatGPT's capacity to generate differential diagnoses, concluding that, while it can aid clinicians, its inconsistent responses limit its potential to replace clinical judgment. Meanwhile, Fraser et al. [51] compared ChatGPT-3.5 and ChatGPT-4 in triage and diagnosis, finding that ChatGPT-3.5 possessed high diagnostic accuracy but insufficient triage abilities. ChatGPT-4 showed improved triaging capability but lower diagnostic accuracy. The authors advised against unsupervised patient use and advocated for efforts to improve diagnostic and triage accuracy. Further studies highlighting ChatGPT's potential in emergency medicine include its role in suggesting diagnostic imaging [52] and providing diagnostic recommendations based on electrocardiography data [53]. Given that hand injuries are often first seen and evaluated in the ED [1,23,54], equipping emergency providers with resources like LLMs can help expedite triage and diagnostic workup.

The potential of LLMs to expedite diagnostic workup and management presents a promising solution for supporting emergency and primary care providers in managing hand injuries rapidly while waiting for a hand surgeon. This application could be especially advantageous in rural or underserved areas lacking on-site hand specialists. LLMs can empower these frontline providers to initiate diagnostic processes and treatment strategies, serving as a valuable resource until a hand specialist can evaluate the patient. This concept of using LLMs as a specialty consult has been previously discussed in the literature [50,51,55,56]. However, it is important to note that, while LLMs can support providers and bridge the gap between the initial presentation and hand surgery evaluation, they should not be used to replace an actual consultation with a hand specialist [1,11,13,24].

4.1. Ethical Considerations

As the integration of LLMs into medical practice becomes increasingly prevalent, it is imperative to address the ethical considerations and limitations associated with their use. While LLMs offer immense potential to enhance patient care and medical decision making in hand surgery, they also pose ethical challenges that necessitate careful attention. Upholding ethical principles, such as autonomy, beneficence, nonmaleficence, and justice, is paramount in the development and deployment of these models.

- Autonomy: Healthcare providers must ensure that LLMs respect a patient's autonomy by facilitating informed decision making and respecting their preferences and values, especially throughout the surgical process [57,58]. A patient's autonomy may be compromised if they are not adequately informed about the limitations, biases, and role of LLMs in their care [1,59].
- Beneficence: LLMs have the potential to significantly benefit patient care by providing timely and accurate information that can empower both healthcare professionals and patients to make more informed decisions. However, the implementation of LLMs must be guided by a commitment to maximizing these potential benefits while minimizing harm [48,59].
- Nonmaleficence: While LLMs can offer valuable assistance, they also carry inherent risks, including the potential for errors, biases, and misinformation [1,3,11,48]. Healthcare providers must critically evaluate and verify LLM-generated recommendations. Additionally, measures should be in place to mitigate the risk of LLMs propagating misinformation or perpetuating bias and healthcare disparities [57,59]. This entails the

ongoing monitoring and evaluation of LLM performance, as well as efforts to address any identified issues or limitations.

- Justice: The fair distribution of resources requires equitable access to this technology and its benefits [2]. Failing to address LLM bias and disparities in LLM utilization could exacerbate existing inequities in healthcare access and outcomes [1,2,52,57]. Therefore, it is imperative for healthcare systems to implement policies and initiatives aimed at promoting equitable access to LLM technology.

By paying careful attention to issues such as data privacy, transparency in decision-making processes, liability, and the mitigation of biases, healthcare can navigate the integration of LLMs in a manner that prioritizes ethical integrity. By proactively addressing these ethical considerations, healthcare can harness the full potential of LLMs while safeguarding patient autonomy, well-being, and justice in medical practice.

4.2. Limitations

We acknowledge multiple limitations to the study and the generalizability of its results. The clinical scenarios depicted in this study adhered closely to textbook examples. This prompts the question: how would these models fare when faced with less straightforward vignettes? Real-life patient encounters frequently involve atypical or complex presentations, which may diverge from the expected norms. Models trained solely on textbook-like cases may struggle to accurately interpret and respond to the complexities inherent in real-world medical practice. Evaluating these models' adaptability to a wide range of clinical scenarios is essential for their effectiveness. Failing to do so risks undermining their reliability and applicability in real-world healthcare settings, potentially compromising patient care outcomes. Therefore, future research endeavors should prioritize testing these models against a wider range of clinical vignettes to comprehensively assess their real-world utility and identify areas for improvement.

Although this study included 68 unique patient vignettes covering 12 classification systems, it is by no means comprehensive. While these vignettes offer valuable insights into the classification abilities of the models under examination, they may not fully encapsulate the diverse spectrum of hand injuries encountered in clinical practice. As such, the study's findings should be interpreted within the context of its inherent constraints. Despite these challenges, our study serves as a starting point for future investigations to delve into these nuances and to advance our understanding of LLM performance in real-world clinical practice.

Furthermore, the success of using LLMs in medicine depends entirely on their ability to provide accurate and reliable information. The speed at which an LLM can respond to queries becomes irrelevant if it offers incorrect and potentially harmful recommendations. Misinformation can lead to adverse patient outcomes and the erosion of trust in technology and healthcare providers [9,57,60]. As previously mentioned, we acknowledge that neither ChatGPT nor Gemini was designed specifically with medical applications in mind. The datasets on which these models were trained likely lack significant medical information and data. This inherent limitation underscores the importance of further refining LLMs specifically for healthcare applications in order to mitigate such shortcomings.

4.3. Future Research and Next Steps

Moving forward, it is imperative to address the limitations highlighted in this study to maximize the potential of LLMs in healthcare. While ChatGPT and Gemini have exhibited promising capabilities in classifying hand injuries and offering management recommendations, there remains a need for further research to refine and enhance their performance for real-world clinical applications. One crucial area of focus for future investigation involves expanding the training datasets of these LLMs with more comprehensive medical information and clinical data. This would allow these models to better navigate the intricacies of medical decision making. Additionally, future studies should aim to evaluate the performance of ChatGPT, Gemini, and other LLMs in classifying atypical or complex hand injuries, as well as extending their assessment to encompass a broader spectrum of injuries and medical conditions. Most current studies focus exclusively on ChatGPT, but with Gemini's superior performance in hand injury classification, further studies examining this model's ability are warranted. By systematically examining LLM performance in diverse clinical scenarios, researchers can identify areas for improvement and tailor these models to address the specific challenges encountered in medical practice.

Furthermore, the advancement of LLMs in medicine necessitates ongoing research and development. By continually refining and validating AI tools like ChatGPT and Gemini, healthcare professionals can harness their full potential as invaluable resources in clinical practice. Further investigation into the use and performance of additional AI tools like RAG, especially when used in conjunction with LLMs, is indicated. Through collaborative interdisciplinary efforts between developers, healthcare institutions, and medical professionals, the development of robust and reliable medical-focused LLMs can pave the way for a new era of personalized and efficient healthcare delivery.

5. Conclusions

This study evaluates the performance of ChatGPT and Gemini in classifying hand injuries and suggesting management. While both models show potential, Gemini generally performs better than ChatGPT in classification, although not currently at a suitable level for current use. For treatment recommendations, ChatGPT leans towards recommending surgical intervention more readily, albeit with lower specificity than Gemini. These findings stress the need to carefully weigh the strengths and limitations of different LLMs when incorporating them into clinical practice. Both ChatGPT and Gemini hold promise as valuable resources for hand surgeons. This potential is expected to translate into enhanced diagnostic accuracy and treatment decisions, ultimately improving patient outcomes. However, further development and research are necessary to ensure the reliability of these models.

Author Contributions: Conceptualization, S.M.P. and A.J.F.; methodology, S.M.P., S.B., C.A.G.-C. and S.A.H.; software, S.M.P., S.B. and A.J.F.; validation, S.M.P. and S.B.; formal analysis, S.M.P.; investigation, S.M.P.; resources, NA; data curation, S.M.P., S.B., C.A.G.-C. and S.A.H.; writing—original draft preparation, S.M.P., S.B., C.A.G.-C. and S.A.H.; writing—review and editing, S.M.P., S.B., C.A.G.-C., S.A.H. and A.J.F.; visualization, S.M.P. and A.J.F.; supervision, A.J.F.; project administration, A.J.F. All authors have read and agreed to the published version of the manuscript.

Funding: This research received no external funding.

Institutional Review Board Statement: Ethical review and approval was not applicable for this study since no patient information was used. Patient scenarios were fictionalized.

Informed Consent Statement: Not applicable.

Data Availability Statement: The data that support the findings of this study are available from the corresponding author upon reasonable request.

Acknowledgments: The authors acknowledge the use of ChatGPT in text editing and the creation of icons for Figure 4. The authors assume full responsibility for the content of this article.

Conflicts of Interest: The authors declare no conflicts of interest.

References

1. Miller, R.; Farnebo, S.; Horwitz, M.D. Insights and trends review: Artificial intelligence in hand surgery. *J. Hand Surg. Eur. Vol.* **2023**, *48*, 396–403. [CrossRef] [PubMed]
2. Topol, E.J. High-performance medicine: The convergence of human and artificial intelligence. *Nat. Med.* **2019**, *25*, 44–56. [CrossRef] [PubMed]
3. Dave, T.; Athaluri, S.A.; Singh, S. ChatGPT in medicine: An overview of its applications, advantages, limitations, future prospects, and ethical considerations. *Front. Artif. Intell.* **2023**, *6*, 1169595. [CrossRef] [PubMed]
4. Ulusoy, I.; Yılmaz, M.; Kıvrak, A. How Efficient Is ChatGPT in Accessing Accurate and Quality Health-Related Information? *Cureus* **2023**, *15*, e46662. [CrossRef] [PubMed]

5. Mikolov, T.; Karafiát, M.; Burget, L.; Cernocký, J.; Khudanpur, S. Recurrent neural network based language model. In *Interspeech*; ISCA: Chiba, Japan, 2010; pp. 1045–1048.
6. Jin, Z. Analysis of the Technical Principles of ChatGPT and Prospects for Pre-trained Large Models. In Proceedings of the 2023 IEEE 3rd International Conference on Information Technology, Big Data and Artificial Intelligence (ICIBA), Chongqing, China, 26–28 May 2023; pp. 1755–1758.
7. Google. Gemini. Available online: https://gemini.google.com/app (accessed on 10 March 2024).
8. OpenAI. ChatGPT. Available online: https://chat.openai.com/chat (accessed on 10 March 2024).
9. Abi-Rafeh, J.; Xu, H.H.; Kazan, R.; Tevlin, R.; Furnas, H. Large Language Models and Artificial Intelligence: A Primer for Plastic Surgeons on the Demonstrated & Potential Applications, Promises, and Limitations of ChatGPT. *Aesthet. Surg. J.* **2023**, *44*, 329–343. [CrossRef] [PubMed]
10. Kung, T.H.; Cheatham, M.; Medenilla, A.; Sillos, C.; De Leon, L.; Elepaño, C.; Madriaga, M.; Aggabao, R.; Diaz-Candido, G.; Maningo, J.; et al. Performance of ChatGPT on USMLE: Potential for AI-assisted medical education using large language models. *PLoS Digit. Health* **2023**, *2*, e0000198. [CrossRef] [PubMed]
11. Ghanem, D.; Nassar, J.; El Bachour, J.; Hanna, T. ChatGPT Earns American Board Certification in Hand Surgery. *Hand Surg. Rehabil.* **2024**, 101688. [CrossRef] [PubMed]
12. Sallam, M. ChatGPT Utility in Healthcare Education, Research, and Practice: Systematic Review on the Promising Perspectives and Valid Concerns. *Healthcare* **2023**, *11*, 887. [CrossRef] [PubMed]
13. Keller, M.; Guebeli, A.; Thieringer, F.; Honigmann, P. Artificial intelligence in patient-specific hand surgery: A scoping review of literature. *Int. J. Comput. Assist. Radiol. Surg.* **2023**, *18*, 1393–1403. [CrossRef]
14. Gummesson, C.; Ward, M.M.; Atroshi, I. The shortened disabilities of the arm, shoulder and hand questionnaire (Quick DASH): Validity and reliability based on responses within the full-length DASH. *BMC Musculoskelet. Disord.* **2006**, *7*, 1–7. [CrossRef]
15. Poerbodipoero, S.; Steultjens, M.; Van der Beek, A.; Dekker, J. Pain, disability in daily activities and work participation in patients with traumatic hand injury. *Br. J. Hand Ther.* **2007**, *12*, 40–47. [CrossRef]
16. Schier, J.S.; Chan, J. Changes in life roles after hand injury. *J. Hand Ther.* **2007**, *20*, 57–69. [CrossRef] [PubMed]
17. Smith, M.E.; Auchincloss, J.M.; Ali, M.S. Causes and consequences of hand injury. *J. Hand Surg. Br.* **1985**, *10*, 288–292. [CrossRef] [PubMed]
18. Angly, B.; Constantinescu, M.A.; Kreutziger, J.; Juon, B.H.; Vögelin, E. Early versus delayed surgical treatment in open hand injuries: A paradigm revisited. *World J. Surg.* **2012**, *36*, 826–829. [CrossRef]
19. del Pinal, F. Severe mutilating injuries to the hand: Guidelines for organizing the chaos. *J. Plast. Reconstr. Aesthet. Surg.* **2007**, *60*, 816–827. [CrossRef] [PubMed]
20. Gustilo, R.B.; Anderson, J.T. Prevention of infection in the treatment of one thousand and twenty-five open fractures of long bones: Retrospective and prospective analyses. *J. Bone Joint Surg. Am.* **1976**, *58*, 453–458. [CrossRef] [PubMed]
21. Salazar Botero, S.; Hidalgo Diaz, J.J.; Benaïda, A.; Collon, S.; Facca, S.; Liverneaux, P.A. Review of Acute Traumatic Closed Mallet Finger Injuries in Adults. *Arch. Plast. Surg.* **2016**, *43*, 134–144. [CrossRef]
22. Wong, K.; von Schroeder, H.P. Delays and Poor Management of Scaphoid Fractures: Factors Contributing to Nonunion. *J. Hand Surg.* **2011**, *36*, 1471–1474. [CrossRef]
23. Yoong, P.; Johnson, C.A.; Yoong, E.; Chojnowski, A. Four hand injuries not to miss: Avoiding pitfalls in the emergency department. *Eur. J. Emerg. Med.* **2011**, *18*, 186–191. [CrossRef] [PubMed]
24. Leypold, T.; Schäfer, B.; Boos, A.; Beier, J.P. Can AI Think Like a Plastic Surgeon? Evaluating GPT-4's Clinical Judgment in Reconstructive Procedures of the Upper Extremity. *Plast. Reconstr. Surg. Glob. Open* **2023**, *11*, e5471. [CrossRef]
25. Crook, B.S.; Park, C.N.; Hurley, E.T.; Richard, M.J.; Pidgeon, T.S. Evaluation of Online Artificial Intelligence-Generated Information on Common Hand Procedures. *J. Hand Surg. Am.* **2023**, *48*, 1122–1127. [CrossRef] [PubMed]
26. Seth, I.; Xie, Y.; Rodwell, A.; Gracias, D.; Bulloch, G.; Hunter-Smith, D.J.; Rozen, W.M. Exploring the Role of a Large Language Model on Carpal Tunnel Syndrome Management: An Observation Study of ChatGPT. *J. Hand Surg. Am.* **2023**, *48*, 1025–1033. [CrossRef] [PubMed]
27. Al Rawi, Z.M.; Kirby, B.J.; Albrecht, P.A.; Nuelle, J.A.V.; London, D.A. Experimenting With the New Frontier: Artificial Intelligence-Powered Chat Bots in Hand Surgery. *Hand* **2024**, 15589447241238372. [CrossRef] [PubMed]
28. Cooney, W.P., 3rd. Scaphoid fractures: Current treatments and techniques. *Instr. Course Lect.* **2003**, *52*, 197–208. [PubMed]
29. Cooney, W.P.; Dobyns, J.H.; Linscheid, R.L. Fractures of the scaphoid: A rational approach to management. *Clin. Orthop. Relat. Res.* **1980**, *149*, 90–97. [CrossRef]
30. Eaton, R.G.; Malerich, M.M. Volar plate arthroplasty of the proximal interphalangeal joint: A review of ten years' experience. *J. Hand Surg. Am.* **1980**, *5*, 260–268. [CrossRef] [PubMed]
31. Geissler, W.B. Arthroscopic management of scapholunate instability. *J. Wrist Surg.* **2013**, *2*, 129–135. [CrossRef] [PubMed]
32. Green, D.P.; O'Brien, E.T. Fractures of the thumb metacarpal. *South. Med. J.* **1972**, *65*, 807–814. [CrossRef] [PubMed]
33. Gustilo, R.B.; Mendoza, R.M.; Williams, D.N. Problems in the management of type III (severe) open fractures: A new classification of type III open fractures. *J. Trauma.* **1984**, *24*, 742–746. [CrossRef] [PubMed]
34. Herbert, T.J.; Fisher, W.E. Management of the fractured scaphoid using a new bone screw. *J. Bone Joint Surg. Br.* **1984**, *66*, 114–123. [CrossRef]

35. Hintermann, B.; Holzach, P.J.; Schütz, M.; Matter, P. Skier's thumb--the significance of bony injuries. *Am. J. Sports Med.* **1993**, *21*, 800–804. [CrossRef] [PubMed]
36. Kleinert, H.E.; Verdan, C. Report of the Committee on Tendon Injuries. *J. Hand Surg.* **1983**, *8*, 794–798. [CrossRef] [PubMed]
37. Leddy, J.P.; Packer, J.W. Avulsion of the profundus tendon insertion in athletes. *J. Hand Surg. Am.* **1977**, *2*, 66–69. [CrossRef]
38. Lichtman, D.M.; Pientka, W.F., 2nd; Bain, G.I. Kienböck Disease: A New Algorithm for the 21st Century. *J. Wrist Surg.* **2017**, *6*, 2–10. [CrossRef] [PubMed]
39. Mayfield, J.K.; Johnson, R.P.; Kilcoyne, R.K. Carpal dislocations: Pathomechanics and progressive perilunar instability. *J. Hand Surg. Am.* **1980**, *5*, 226–241. [CrossRef]
40. Carlà, M.M.; Gambini, G.; Baldascino, A.; Boselli, F.; Giannuzzi, F.; Margollicci, F.; Rizzo, S. Large language models as assistance for glaucoma surgical cases: A ChatGPT vs. Google Gemini comparison. *Graefes Arch. Clin. Exp. Ophthalmol.* **2024**. [CrossRef] [PubMed]
41. Carlà, M.M.; Gambini, G.; Baldascino, A.; Giannuzzi, F.; Boselli, F.; Crincoli, E.; D'Onofrio, N.C.; Rizzo, S. Exploring AI-chatbots' capability to suggest surgical planning in ophthalmology: ChatGPT versus Google Gemini analysis of retinal detachment cases. *Br. J. Ophthalmol.* **2024**. [CrossRef]
42. Koga, S.; Martin, N.B.; Dickson, D.W. Evaluating the performance of large language models: ChatGPT and Google Bard in generating differential diagnoses in clinicopathological conferences of neurodegenerative disorders. *Brain Pathol.* **2023**, *34*, e13207. [CrossRef] [PubMed]
43. Kumari, A.; Kumari, A.; Singh, A.; Singh, S.K.; Juhi, A.; Dhanvijay, A.K.D.; Pinjar, M.J.; Mondal, H. Large Language Models in Hematology Case Solving: A Comparative Study of ChatGPT-3.5, Google Bard, and Microsoft Bing. *Cureus* **2023**, *15*, e43861. [CrossRef]
44. Lim, Z.W.; Pushpanathan, K.; Yew, S.M.E.; Lai, Y.; Sun, C.H.; Lam, J.S.H.; Chen, D.Z.; Goh, J.H.L.; Tan, M.C.J.; Sheng, B.; et al. Benchmarking large language models' performances for myopia care: A comparative analysis of ChatGPT-3.5, ChatGPT-4.0, and Google Bard. *EBioMedicine* **2023**, *95*, 104770. [CrossRef]
45. Rahsepar, A.A.; Tavakoli, N.; Kim, G.H.J.; Hassani, C.; Abtin, F.; Bedayat, A. How AI Responds to Common Lung Cancer Questions: ChatGPT vs Google Bard. *Radiology* **2023**, *307*, e230922. [CrossRef] [PubMed]
46. Gan, R.K.; Ogbodo, J.C.; Wee, Y.Z.; Gan, A.Z.; González, P.A. Performance of Google bard and ChatGPT in mass casualty incidents triage. *Am. J. Emerg. Med.* **2024**, *75*, 72–78. [CrossRef] [PubMed]
47. Zúñiga Salazar, G.; Zúñiga, D.; Vindel, C.L.; Yoong, A.M.; Hincapie, S.; Zúñiga, A.B.; Zúñiga, P.; Salazar, E.; Zúñiga, B. Efficacy of AI Chats to Determine an Emergency: A Comparison Between OpenAI's ChatGPT, Google Bard, and Microsoft Bing AI Chat. *Cureus* **2023**, *15*, e45473. [CrossRef]
48. Berg, H.T.; van Bakel, B.; van de Wouw, L.; Jie, K.E.; Schipper, A.; Jansen, H.; O'Connor, R.D.; van Ginneken, B.; Kurstjens, S. ChatGPT and Generating a Differential Diagnosis Early in an Emergency Department Presentation. *Ann. Emerg. Med.* **2024**, *83*, 83–86. [CrossRef] [PubMed]
49. Franc, J.M.; Cheng, L.; Hart, A.; Hata, R.; Hertelendy, A. Repeatability, reproducibility, and diagnostic accuracy of a commercial large language model (ChatGPT) to perform emergency department triage using the Canadian triage and acuity scale. *Cjem* **2024**, *26*, 40–46. [CrossRef] [PubMed]
50. Funk, P.F.; Hoch, C.C.; Knoedler, S.; Knoedler, L.; Cotofana, S.; Sofo, G.; Bashiri Dezfouli, A.; Wollenberg, B.; Guntinas-Lichius, O.; Alfertshofer, M. ChatGPT's Response Consistency: A Study on Repeated Queries of Medical Examination Questions. *Eur. J. Investig. Health Psychol. Educ.* **2024**, *14*, 657–668. [CrossRef]
51. Fraser, H.; Crossland, D.; Bacher, I.; Ranney, M.; Madsen, T.; Hilliard, R. Comparison of Diagnostic and Triage Accuracy of Ada Health and WebMD Symptom Checkers, ChatGPT, and Physicians for Patients in an Emergency Department: Clinical Data Analysis Study. *JMIR Mhealth Uhealth* **2023**, *11*, e49995. [CrossRef] [PubMed]
52. Barash, Y.; Klang, E.; Konen, E.; Sorin, V. ChatGPT-4 Assistance in Optimizing Emergency Department Radiology Referrals and Imaging Selection. *J. Am. Coll. Radiol.* **2023**, *20*, 998–1003. [CrossRef] [PubMed]
53. Günay, S.; Öztürk, A.; Özerol, H.; Yiğit, Y.; Erenler, A.K. Comparison of emergency medicine specialist, cardiologist, and chat-GPT in electrocardiography assessment. *Am. J. Emerg. Med.* **2024**, *80*, 51–60. [CrossRef]
54. van Leerdam, R.H.; Krijnen, P.; Panneman, M.J.; Schipper, I.B. Incidence and treatment of hand and wrist injuries in Dutch emergency departments. *Eur. J. Trauma. Emerg. Surg.* **2022**, *48*, 4327–4332. [CrossRef]
55. Rizwan, A.; Sadiq, T. The Use of AI in Diagnosing Diseases and Providing Management Plans: A Consultation on Cardiovascular Disorders With ChatGPT. *Cureus* **2023**, *15*, e43106. [CrossRef] [PubMed]
56. Sun, Y.X.; Li, Z.M.; Huang, J.Z.; Yu, N.Z.; Long, X. GPT-4: The Future of Cosmetic Procedure Consultation? *Aesthet. Surg. J.* **2023**, *43*, NP670–NP672. [CrossRef] [PubMed]
57. Oleck, N.C.; Naga, H.I.; Nichols, D.S.; Morris, M.X.; Dhingra, B.; Patel, A. Navigating the Ethical Landmines of ChatGPT: Implications of Intelligent Chatbots in Plastic Surgery Clinical Practice. *Plast. Reconstr. Surg. Glob. Open* **2023**, *11*, e5290. [CrossRef] [PubMed]
58. Pressman, S.M.; Borna, S.; Gomez-Cabello, C.A.; Haider, S.A.; Haider, C.; Forte, A.J. AI and Ethics: A Systematic Review of the Ethical Considerations of Large Language Model Use in Surgery Research. *Healthcare* **2024**, *12*, 825. [CrossRef] [PubMed]

59. Keskinbora, K.H. Medical ethics considerations on artificial intelligence. *J. Clin. Neurosci.* **2019**, *64*, 277–282. [CrossRef]
60. Li, W.; Zhang, Y.; Chen, F. ChatGPT in Colorectal Surgery: A Promising Tool or a Passing Fad? *Ann. Biomed. Eng.* **2023**, *51*, 1892–1897. [CrossRef]

Journal of
Clinical Medicine

MDPI

Article

Is the Tendon-to-Groove Ratio Associated with Elevated Risk for LHB Tendon Disorders?—A New Approach of Preoperative MR-Graphic Analysis for Targeted Diagnosis of Tendinopathy of the Long Head of Biceps

Kristina Gerhardinger [1], Lisa Klute [2], Christian Pfeifer [2,3], Josina Straub [2], Laura Hechinger [2], Moritz Riedl [2], Volker Alt [2], Maximilian Kerschbaum [2] and Leopold Henssler [2,*]

1 Department of Trauma Surgery, Orthopaedics and Sports Medicine, Hospital Barmherzige Brueder, 93049 Regensburg, Germany
2 Department of Trauma Surgery, University Hospital Regensburg, 93053 Regensburg, Germany
3 Department of Trauma and Hand Surgery, Innklinikum Altötting, 84503 Altötting, Germany
* Correspondence: leopold.henssler@ukr.de

Abstract: Background: Pathologies of the long head of the biceps (LHB) tendon are a common cause of anterior shoulder pain. While the influence of the anatomical morphology of the intertubercular groove (ITG) on the development of LHB tendon instability has been investigated with ambiguous results, the relationship of the LHB to ITG anatomy has not yet been considered in this context. The objective of this study was to reliably extract the tendon-to-groove ratio from MRI scans of symptomatic patients and examine its potential influence on the occurrence of certain causes for LHB-associated symptoms. **Methods**: In this retrospective study, preoperative MRI scans of 35 patients (mean age of 46 ± 14 years) presenting with anterior shoulder pain and clinical indications of LHB tendinopathy were analyzed in transversal planes. Long and short diameters of the LHB tendon and ITG were measured, cross-sectional areas of the LHB tendon and ITG were calculated from these measurements, and the ratio of cross-sectional areas (LHB/ITG) was introduced. All measurements were repeated independently by three investigators and inter-rater reliability was assessed using intraclass correlation coefficient (ICC). Thereafter, tendon-to-groove ratios were compared in patients with and without intraoperative signs of LHB tendon instability. **Results**: All patients exhibited intraoperative signs of LHB tendinitis, with additional findings including pulley lesions and SLAP lesions. Analysis revealed variations in the dimensions of the LHB tendon and ITG cross sections, with the tendon-to-groove ratio decreasing from 37% at the pulley to 31% at the deepest point of the sulcus. Very good inter-rater reliability was observed for all measurements. The tendon-to-groove ratio did not significantly differ ($p > 0.05$) in patients with or without pulley lesions or SLAP lesions. **Conclusions**: Our study introduced the novel parameter of the tendon-to-groove ratio of cross-sectional areas as a reproducible parameter for the description of local anatomy in the field of targeted diagnosis of LHB tendon disorders. While our findings do not yet support the predictive value of the tendon-to-groove ratio, they underscore the importance of further research with larger cohorts and control groups to validate these observations.

Keywords: shoulder; biceps tendon; intertubercular groove; arthroscopy; pulley lesions

1. Introduction

Pathologies of the long head of the biceps (LHB) tendon are a common cause of anterior shoulder pain [1]. In over 75% of arthroscopic surgeries of the shoulder, concomitant pathologies of the LHB tendon can be found [2], which require treatment. In addition, the number of arthroscopic biceps tenodesis procedures has constantly increased over the past decade because the field of indications has widened [3–5]. Common pathologies of the LHB tendon include tendinitis, tenosynovitis, subluxation, dislocation, and tears [6,7]. These conditions often manifest as anterior shoulder pain, weakness, and clicking sensations during arm movements. While tendinitis and tenosynovitis typically result from overuse or degeneration, subluxation and dislocation can occur due to instability of the biceps tendon within the intertubercular groove (ITG) [7–10]. Tears of the LHB tendon may occur acutely due to trauma or as a result of degenerative changes. These pathologies can significantly impair shoulder function and quality of life, necessitating prompt diagnosis and appropriate management strategies [5,10].

Originating from the supraglenoid tubercle and partly from the superior glenoid labrum, which is summarized as the SLAP (superior labrum from anterior to posterior) complex, the LHB tendon resides intra-articularly but extrasynovially, encompassed by a synovial-lined sheath extending into the ITG [3,6]. Proximal to the intertubercular groove the coracohumeral ligament and superior glenohumeral ligament fuse along the lateral half of the rotator interval with fibers from the subscapularis and supraspinatus tendons to form the biceps reflection pulley—a sling-like structure stabilizing the long head of the biceps tendon [11,12] at its entry to the intertubercular groove. Upon passing the biceps reflection pulley, the LHB tendon undergoes a 30- to 40-degree angulation as it enters the intertubercular groove [3,13]. The integrity of the tendon's fixation system of the SLAP complex and biceps pulley system is crucial since instability of the LHB tendon may not only lead to painful LHB tendinitis but also can cause rotator cuff lesions [7,10,14].

From a physiological viewpoint, it is certain that the resultant force vector, that builds up during arm loading, varies—in certain glenohumeral positions, it may point directly into the intertubercular groove, stabilizing the tendon, whereas in other positions, the tendon may directly load the pulley reflection complex, potentially causing instability or injury [13]. Thus, due to LHB instability, e.g., caused by pulley lesions, the tendon gets successively damaged by moving over the tuberosities sideways during rotation of the arm [7].

At the same time, lesions of the biceps pulley system are sometimes difficult to detect on preoperative MR imaging unless there is a subluxation of the tendon. Therefore, it would be helpful for treating physicians to look for indirect signs or predisposing anatomical conditions in patients suffering from LHB-related symptoms without clear evidence of structural damage in MR imaging.

Anatomical variations in the size, depth, and configuration of the intertubercular groove may also influence force vectors and the likelihood of LHB instability [7,15–18]. Consequently, the presence of certain anatomical features reliably assessable in pre-operative MR imaging, could serve as indicators for present LHB tendon pathologies [19,20].

Different morphological configurations of the ITG have already been the subject of numerous investigations as possible predispositions for the development of an instability of the LHB tendon, coming to different results [16,21,22].

However, to the authors' knowledge, there is no study that examines the influence of the LHB tendon's dimensions and, in particular, its dimensions in relation to the dimensions of the intertubercular groove. To consider only the individual ITG anatomy in the individual predisposition to instability and to disregard the different dimensions of the LHB tendon represents a very one-sided and therefore incomplete view of the interaction of the two anatomical structures affected.

Therefore, the objective of this study was to examine the morphology of the ITG and long head of biceps tendon, including the cross-sectional areas of the LHB tendon and ITG and to assess whether the tendon-to-groove ratio can be reliably extracted from preoperative MRI scans by different examiners.

The second objective was to assess whether this new parameter may be valuable as a prognostic factor for structural LHB tendon disease that could aid in clinical decision making or targeted patient treatment.

2. Materials and Methods

2.1. Study Cohort

Data were obtained from MRI scans of the shoulder region of patients who presented at our outpatient department due to acute or degenerative injuries affecting the rotator cuff or labroligamentous structures of the shoulder. Inclusion criteria encompassed the presence of concurrent anterior shoulder pain and clinical indications of biceps tendinopathy upon examination, age exceeding 18 years, and MRI scans conducted at our institution. Exclusion criteria comprised MRI scans obtained from external institutions, diagnoses of inflammatory arthritis or advanced osteoarthritis, and a history of significant trauma or previous open/arthroscopic surgeries on the affected shoulder (Figure 1). Approval from the institutional ethics review board was obtained prior to the commencement of this study (number: 18-1032-101).

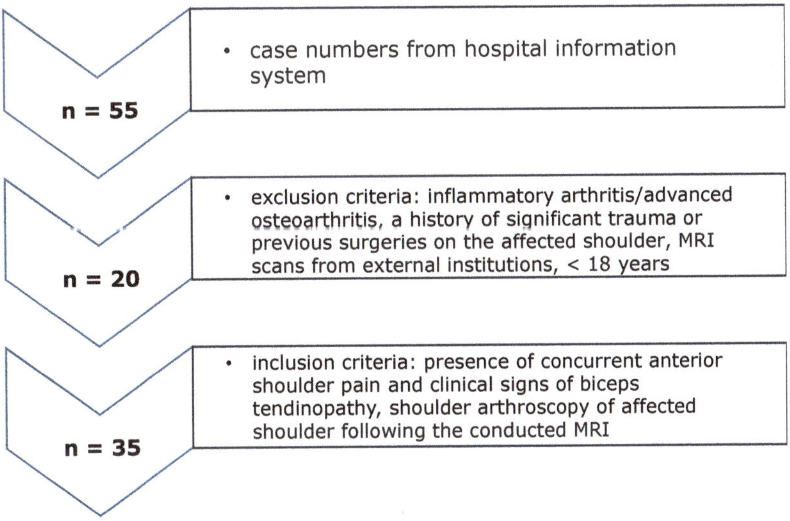

Figure 1. Inclusion and exclusion criteria of the study cohort.

2.2. MRI Measurements

Patients were positioned in a closed MRI scanner (MAGNETOM Skyra, Siemens Healthineers AG, Forchheim, Germany) in the supine position, with the upper extremity placed alongside the body, the elbow fully extended, and the forearm in a neutral rotation. All MRI scans were conducted utilizing the same scanner. Standard shoulder sequences were executed using a specialized shoulder coil, incorporating proton density (PD) sequences for acquiring images in the axial plane (repetition time/echo time (TR/TE) range: 3000–3220/33 ms; section thickness: 3 mm; field of view: 15 cm), which were of primary interest for this investigation. Image analysis was performed utilizing the syngo PACS viewer (Siemens Healthineers AG, Forchheim, Germany). The positioning of the long head of the biceps tendon in relation to the entire length of the intertubercular groove was evaluated on axial PD-weighted images, with measurements taken both at the entrance of the intertubercular groove (measuring point 1) and at its deepest point (measuring point 2).

Specific dimensions and angles were gathered for the analysis of the anatomy of the long head of the biceps tendon and the intertubercular groove in the MRI scans (Figures 2 and 3):

1. Long axis of the elliptical LHB tendon cross-section (Figure 2a);
2. Short axis of the elliptical LHB tendon cross-section (Figure 2b);
3. Depth of the ITG (Figure 2d);

4. Width of the ITG (Figure 2e);
5. Medial wall angle (MWA, Figure 3a);
6. Adapted opening angle (AOA, Figure 3b).

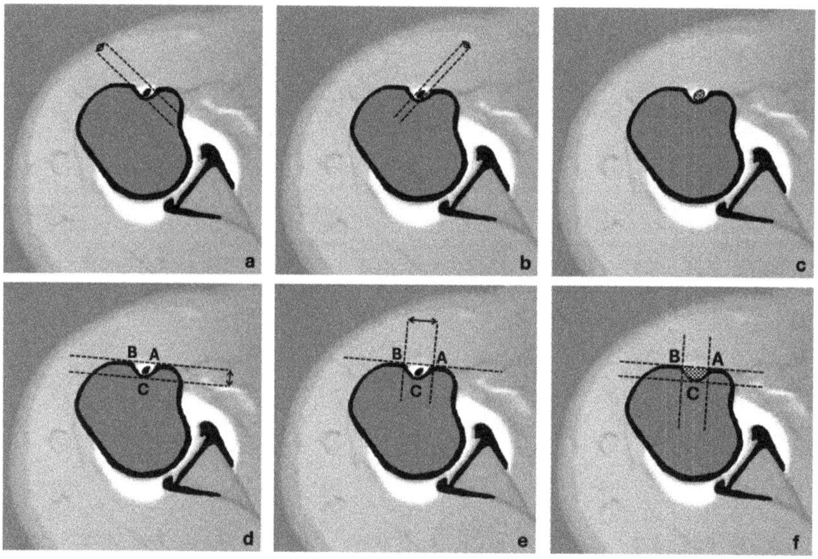

Figure 2. Dimensions that were extracted from axial PD images at both measuring points: Long axis of the LHB tendon (**a**) and short axis of the LHB tendon (**b**). For the measurement of the dimensions of the ITG various straight lines and points were defined: First, a straight line was created that was tangent to both edges of the ITG. The point of contact of the tangent at the lesser tuberosity was labeled A and the point of contact at the greater tuberosity was labeled B. A second parallel straight line was then drawn and shifted in parallel so that it was tangent to the deepest point of the ITB. The point of contact of the second tangent with the base of the ITG was labeled C. The depth of the ITG was measured as the distance between the two straight lines (**d**). The distance between points A and B was used to measure the width of the ITG (**e**) and depth of the ITG (**d**); the cross-sectional areas of both the LHB tendon (**c**) and the ITG (**f**) were calculated from the above measurements.

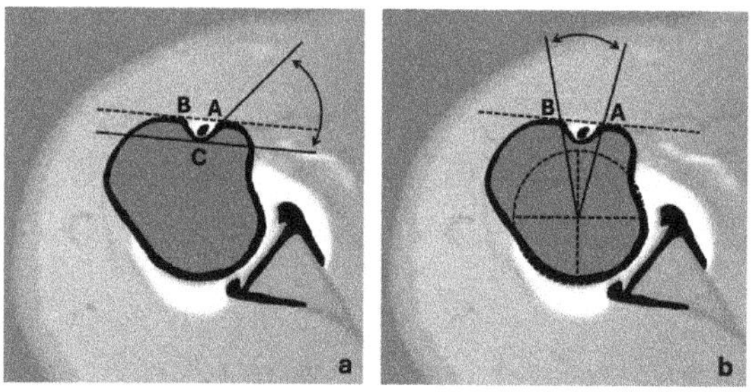

Figure 3. The medial wall angle (MWA, **a**) was determined by measuring the angle formed between a straight-line connecting points A and B and a second line intersecting points A and C. This measurement indicates the inclination of the medial wall of the ITG as it transitions towards the lesser tuberosity. The adapted opening angle (AOA, **b**) was assessed as an angle originating from the center of the best-fit circle of the humeral head and extending from point A to point B. This angle provides information about the degree of opening from the center of the humeral head to the indicated points.

The cross-sectional area of the ITG was calculated under the assumption of a semi-elliptical shape ($A = \pi \times 0.5w \times d \times 0.5$), utilizing the measured dimensions of width (w) and depth (d) as seen in Figure 4. Similarly, the cross-sectional area of the LHB tendon was calculated ($A = \pi \times 0.5w \times 0.5d$) based on the gathered measurements.

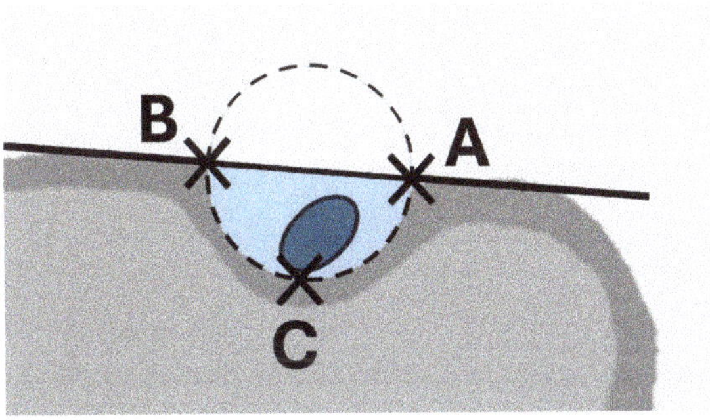

Figure 4. Visualization of the area ratio between the LHB tendon and the intertubercular grove. While the cross-sectional area of the LHB tendon is calculated under the assumption of an elliptic tendon shape (dark blue), the area of the groove was calculated under the assumption of a half-elliptic shape (light blue). Both cross-sectional areas (A–C) were calculated as explained in Figure 2.

Three independent observers (experienced shoulder surgeons) conducted a review of the axial PD slices from each shoulder MRI scan. The examiners were instructed to measure the long and short axis of the tendon and groove anatomy both at the entrance to the ITG and at the deepest point of the ITG. To ensure a high degree of reproducibility and comparability of the measurements, the examiners had visual instructions for the measurements to be determined shown in Figures 2 and 3. All reviewers were blinded to the patients' clinical data and conducted all measurements on their own without knowledge of the other examiners data.

2.3. Statistical Methods

The normality of the data was assessed using Shapiro–Wilk testing, revealing a normal distribution for all measured parameters. However, the calculated parameters, including cross-sectional areas and ratios of cross-sectional areas, did not exhibit a normal distribution. Consequently, continuous data were analyzed and expressed as the mean and standard deviation for normally distributed data, while the median and interquartile range (IQR) were used for non-normally distributed data. Categorical data were presented as total count and percentage. Chi-squared tests were utilized for comparing categorical data, and group comparisons for continuous data were performed using the Mann–Whitney *U* Test for non-normally distributed variables and two-sided *t* test for normally distributed parameters. Inter-rater reliability was expressed with the intraclass correlation coefficient (ICC). Statistical analyses were conducted using IBM SPSS Statistics Version 29 (IBM Inc., Armonk, NY, USA), with significance set at $p < 0.05$.

3. Results

3.1. Patient Collective

We included 35 patients (30 males, 85.7%) with a mean age of 46 ± 14 years (19–73 years). All patients showed intraoperative signs of tendinitis of the LHB tendon. A total of 14 patients (40.0%) were intraoperatively diagnosed with rotator cuff tears, 5 of them with anterosuperior lesions and concomitant lesions of the biceps reflection pulley. Four additional patients (11.4%) showed isolated pulley lesions (PL) without major injury of the rotator cuff. Other intraoperative findings indicating the need for LHB tenodesis were SLAP lesions (6/35 patients, 17.1%) and partial ruptures of the intraarticular portion (5/35 patients, 14.3%).

3.2. Anatomy of the LHB Tendon

The long diameter of the LHB tendon (6.6 ± 2.0 mm) decreased from the entrance of the sulcus (measuring point I) to the deepest point of the sulcus (measuring point II, 6.0 ± 1.4 mm; $p = 0.009$). In contrast, the shorter diameter of the LHB tendon increased in its course and amounted to 2.2 ± 0.6 mm at the sulcus entrance and 2.7 ± 0.5 mm in the middle ITG ($p < 0.001$). Thus, the aspect ratio of the short to the long axis was calculated to a median of 31% (IQR 28–42%) at the pulley and 43% (IQR 39–52%) in the deep ITG. The cross-sectional area of the LHB tendon was calculated from the single measurements and amounted to a median of 9.8 mm^2 (IQR 8.0–14.9 mm^2) at the pulley complex and 12.5 mm^2 (IQR 9.5–14.5 mm^2) at the second measuring point at the deepest point.

All the measurements of the long axis of the tendon (ICC 0.999), short axis of the tendon (ICC 0.991), and the LHB cross-sectional area showed very good inter-rater reliability (ICC 0.995).

Summing up these results, the cross-sectional area of the LHB tendon did not undergo statistically significant changes ($p = 0.232$), even if the changes in the ratio of the short to long axis indicate a change in the shape of the LHB tendon from a relatively flat and oval shape of the intraarticular portion at the pulley complex to a significantly rounder shape of the tendon ($p < 0.001$) over the course through the bicipital groove.

The LHB tendon's dimensions did not significantly differ in patients with and without lesions of the SLAP complex or pulley system (see Table 1).

Table 1. Measures and calculated parameters depending on the presence or absence of pulley lesions or SLAP lesions. LHB = long head of biceps; ITG = intertubercular groove; MWA = medial wall angle; and AOA = adapted opening angle.

	Pulley Lesion			SLAP Lesion		
	No (n = 26)	**Yes (n = 9)**	*p*	**No (n = 29)**	**Yes (n = 6)**	*p*
Measuring point 1 (pulley complex)						
Long tendon diameter (mm)	6.5 ± 1.8	7.0 ± 2.5	0.546 *	6.7 ± 2.1	6.1 ± 1.6	0.520 *
Short tendon diameter (mm)	2.2 ± 0.6	2.2 ± 0.6	0.891 *	2.2 ± 0.6	2.2 ± 0.6	0.793 *
LHB Ratio short diameter/long diameter (%)	30 (IQR 28–42)	35 (IQR 30–40)	0.590 **	31 (IQR 28–42)	30 (IQR 28–35)	0.782 **
Cross-sectional area LHB (mm^2)	9.6 (IQR 8.2–15.6)	11.3 (IQR 8.0–11.8)	0.985 **	10.2 (IQR 8.2–14.3)	9.5 (IQR 8.0–14.9)	0.685 **
ITG width (mm)	11.0 ± 1.5	11.0 ± 1.5	0.961 *	11.2 ± 1.5	10.4 ± 0.9	0.267 *
ITG depth (mm)	3.5 ± 0.8	3.3 ± 0.7	0.456 *	3.4 ± 0.8	4.0 ± 0.8	0.078 *
Cross-sectional area ITG (mm^2)	28.8 (IQR 25.2–36.7)	31.7 (IQR 24.3–35.4)	0.725 **	27.9 (IQR 24.4–35.4)	33.7 (IQR 29.7–39.5)	0.272 **
Ratio LHB/ITG (%)	37 (IQR 25–49)	37 (IQR 31–54)	0.725 **	31 (IQR 28–42)	30 (IQR 28–35)	0.454 **
Measuring point 2 (deepest ITG)						
Long tendon diameter (mm)	5.9 ± 1.4	6.1 ± 1.7	0.817 *	5.9 ± 1.5	6.1 ± 0.8	0.751 *
Short tendon diameter (mm)	2.5 ± 0.5	2.7 ± 0.4	0.464 *	2.6 ± 0.6	2.5 ± 0.4	0.712 *
LHB Ratio short diameter/long diameter (%)	42 (IQR 38–52)	45 (IQR 41–49)	0.697 **	45 (IQR 40–52)	39 (IQR 38–42)	0.218 **
Cross-sectional area LHB (mm^2)	11.7 (IQR 9.0–14.5)	12.8 (IQR 10.2–13.2)	0.540 **	12.5 (IQR 9.7–14.5)	11.9 (IQR 9.5–13.1)	0.983 **
ITG width (mm)	10.4 ± 1.6	10.8 ± 2.7	0.651 *	10.7 ± 1.9	9.4 ± 1.7	0.106 *
ITG depth (mm)	4.9 ± 0.5	4.8 ± 0.5	0.609 *	4.9 ± 0.5	5.1 ± 0.7	0.260 *
Cross-sectional area ITG (mm^2)	39.1 (IQR 32.2–47.4)	42.4 (IQR 35.7–46.1)	0.540 **	41.4 (IQR 32.2–47.4)	35.9 (IQR 35.7–41.9)	0.983 **
Ratio LHB/ITG (%)	33 (IQR 23–38)	28 (IQR 22–38)	0.985 **	30 (IQR 22–38)	33 (IQR 25–35)	0.815 **
MWA (°)	44.8 ± 6.1	47.5 ± 9.7	0.443 *	44.8 ± 6.7	48.9 ± 8.6	0.201 *
AOA (°)	21.2 ± 3.5	21.6 ± 4.6	0.833 *	21.8 ± 3.9	19.1 ± 2.0	0.117 *

* = calculated using independent *t* test; ** = calculated using Mann–Whitney *U* test.

3.3. Anatomy of the Intertubercular Groove

The average dimensions of the intertubercular grove were 11.0 ± 1.5 mm in width and 3.5 ± 0.8 mm in depth at the entrance to the intertubercular grove. At its deepest point, the width of the ITG did not change significantly (10.5 ± 1.9 mm; $p = 0.081$) but the depth increased to 4.9 ± 0.5 mm ($p < 0.001$).

Accordingly, the cross-sectional area of the ITG increased from a median of 29.7 mm^2 (IQR 24.4–36.7 mm^2) at measuring point I to a median of 39.3 mm^2 (IQR 32.4–47.4 mm^2) at measuring point II ($p < 0.001$). We found very good inter-rater reliability for measurements of the ITG width (ICC 0.998) and ITC depth (ICC 0.995) and cross-sectional area of the ITG (ICC 0.996), respectively.

The medial wall angle (MWA) and the adapted opening angle (AOA) measured an average of 45.5 ± 7.1° and 21.3 ± 3.7°, respectively.

Moreover, none of the above mentioned ITG dimensions and angles significantly differed in patients with and without SLAP or pulley lesions (see Table 1).

3.4. The LHB-Tendon-to-Intertubercular-Groove Ratio

The tendon-to-groove ratio of LHB/ITG was determined with very-high inter-rater reliability (ICC 0.991).

Since the cross-sectional area of the LHB tendon over the course from the joint through the ITG remained unchanged and, at the same time, the cross-sectional area of the ITG increased from entrance to deepest point of the ITG, the tendon-to-groove ratio decreased over the tendons course.

The median tendon-to-groove ratio of the cross-sectional areas (LHB/ITG) was significantly higher (37% [IQR 25–54%]) at the pulley complex compared to the ratio at the deepest point of the ITG (31% [IQR 22–38%]; $p = 0.005$).

Neither the ratio of cross-sectional areas nor any of the other measurements or the calculated parameters showed significant differences depending on the presence or absence of a pulley or SLAP lesion (Table 1).

4. Discussion

In our study, dimensions of the long head of biceps tendon and the intertubercular groove were assessed by three independent examiners using preoperative MRI in neutral arm position in patients with anterior shoulder pain and intraoperative signs of tendinitis of the LHB tendon.

Key findings of the study were as follows:

1. The tendon-to-groove ratio of cross-sectional areas was introduced as a new parameter of local anatomy and showed very-high inter-rater reliability;
2. The cross-sectional area ratio of LHB tendon to intertubercular groove decreased from 37% to 31% over its course from the biceps pulley system to the deepest point of the ITG;
3. Neither at measuring point 1 nor at measuring point 2 did the LHB/ITG ratio differ in patients with vs. without pulley lesions or SLAP lesions.

4.1. Intertubercular Groove Morphology and Its Influence on LHB Instability

Many previous studies have focused on certain anatomical configurations of the ITG and their effect on LHB tendon instability and thus higher likelihood of tendinopathy. The current state of knowledge of the available studies on this topic suggests that the depth or width of the groove alone do not play important roles in the pathogenesis of tendon instability but rather the morphology in its entirety. Therefore, the medial wall angle as well as the total opening angle are commonly used parameters to quantify the anatomy of the intertubercular groove. Therefore, all of these parameters were also evaluated in our study to ensure comparability to existing literature.

The depth of the intertubercular groove at its deepest point of 4.9 ± 0.5 mm (measuring point 2) in our cohort complies with results of similar studies. Abboud et al., for example, also assessed MR imaging, measuring a median depth of 5.1 ± 1.97 mm, and Shah et al. found a depth of 5.1 mm in a group of patients with LHBT pathology in comparison to a depth of 5.5 mm in a healthy control group [21,23]. Kavak et al. assessed the depth of the ITG in patients with unstable LHB tendons as well as in patients with stable LHB tendons [24]. The ones with unstable tendons showed an average depth of 5.47 ± 0.23 mm which was also concordant with the results of our study. The healthy control group in the study showed deeper grooves (5.90 ± 0.21 mm) [24]. Looking at the width of the ITG, investigating X-rays of 37 patients with anterior shoulder pain and comparing the results to those of a control group, Pfahler et al. measured a depth of 11.6 mm on average. This is also concordant with the results of the present study which measured 11.0 ± 1.5 mm at the cranial entrance to the ITG (measuring point 1) as well as at the measuring point at maximal ITG depth (measuring point 2) [22].

Contrarily, the mean MWA of 45.5 ± 7.1° measured in the present study diverges almost 10 degrees from the angle Kavak et al. published in 2019 even though they measured the MWA at the deepest point of the ITG using the same reference points as in our study [24]. Kavak et al. showed generally higher angles in patients with stable as well as unstable LHB tendons, with an MWA of 54.66 ± 0.60° and 52.16 ± 0.44°, respectively. Kavaks results resemble the ones of Ulucakoy's study, that showed 49.9 ± 8.4° in the group with unstable LHBT and 51.0 ± 8.6° in a healthy reference group [24,25]. In contrast, the MWA that Shah or Pfahler et al. measured complied well with the ones of the present study, only differing by 2° and 3°, respectively [22,23].

All of these existing investigations are based on the physiological assumption that a deeper groove results in better stabilization of the LHB tendon due to better guidance by the bony walls of the ITG. In 2017, Yoo et al. showed that a shallow intertubercular groove, identified by a larger opening angle, smaller medial angle, and shallower depth may represent a predisposing factor for LHB tendon instability [26]. More than a decade earlier, Spritzer et al. already postulated a strong correlation between ITG morphology and LHB tendon instabilities [27], limited by a small group size and lack of statistical analysis. Taking a closer look at LHB tendon instability and possible subsequent pathologies, Kleim et al. analyzed different types of biceps reflection pulley (BRP) lesions on the basis of arthroscopy findings and showed that lateral BRP injuries are not influenced by the ITG morphology, whilst medial and bilateral ones are [28]. They presumed that a shallow BG morphology may lead to a dislocation of the LHBT, which may move out of the BG medially or laterally while external or internal rotation movement of the humerus subsequently damages the medial or lateral BRP [28]. Looking at this "Skipping" of the LHB tendon out of the ITG, while rubbing over its rims from a pathophysiological viewpoint, it seems at least possible that the LHB tendon itself has a high probability of getting altered or inflamed the more often this dislocation occurs. This hypothesis aligns well with Lafosse et al.'s finding that lesions of the LHB tendon occur significantly more frequently in patients with unstable tendons [7]. In contrast to all the above findings, Abboud et al. did not find any correlation between the medial wall angle or depth of the intertubercular groove and the presence of biceps tendon pathologies during arthroscopy in a study involving 75 patients, conducted with the intention to explore the relationship between ITG morphology and LHB tendon pathologies [21]. Furthermore, Ulucakoy et al. showed that a control group with stable LHB tendons had shallower ITGs with bigger opening angles than the other group with proven LHB tendon instability, concluding that the morphology of the ITG is not related to LHB tendon stability [25].

In summary, the literature on the relationship between the anatomical variants of the ITG and the occurrence of LHB instability is inconclusive. However, it is striking that all of the above-mentioned studies only examine the morphology of the groove, but none of the above studies took the influence of LHB tendon dimensions into account.

Since the dimensions of the tendon can be subject to significant changes over the course of a lifetime due to irritation, associated edematous swelling, paratendinitis, or

chronic mucoid degeneration, the authors believe that a one-sided view of a bilateral problem of instability is too imprecise.

The aim of this present study was, therefore, to investigate the dimensions of both the LHB tendon and the ITG and introduce a parameter that represents the relationship between these two dimensions. For this purpose, the ratio of the cross-sectional areas of tendon-to-groove seemed to be a promising parameter, since it is conceivable that a relatively large tendon in a relatively shallow sulcus could have a higher probability of dislocation. With a corresponding injury mechanism, in which the force vector is acting on the tendon points medially, such an anatomical combination could predispose the development of a medial subluxation.

4.2. Cross-Sectional Areas and LHB/ITG Ratio

The presented study is the first one to assess cross-sectional areas of both the LHB tendon as well as the intertubercular groove in patients with proven LHB tendinitis. To our knowledge, the literature on these anatomical dimensions at different measuring points is very limited.

There is just one study that can be used as a reference for the cross-sectional area of the ITG: Cardoso et al. determined the cross-sectional area at the point of the ITG with maximum depth, which is equivalent to our measuring point 2. Regarding the cohort of 37 patients with LHB tendon pathology, the cross-sectional area of the ITG was 19.1 ± 7.1 mm^2. The healthy control group showed a cross-sectional area of 16.6 ± 4.5 mm^2 [29]. The authors summarized that even though the cross-sectional area width and depth of the ITG were gradually higher in patients with LHB tendon pathology, their study did not support any correlation between LHB tendon pathology and ITG morphology [29].

The results of both groups differ a lot from the cross-sectional area of 29.7 mm^2 that we calculated at the equivalent measuring point. Reasons for this difference of more than 10 mm^2 could either be that the measured dimensions of the groove included in the calculation differ or that Cardoso et al. used a different approximation formula for calculating the cross-sectional area. Either way, even small differences in the variables involved have a major impact on the result, as the formula contains an exponentiation.

Moreover, for the abovementioned rationale, the present study did not only assess the cross-sectional areas of the intertubercular groove and the LHB tendon but put both to a relation. However, no difference of the new parameter could be found in patients with or without structural lesions of the LHB tendon's fixation points.

Even if further studies may be able to show a predictive value of the LHB/ITG ratio for present pathological alterations of the LHB, it has to be defined which clinical implications can be drawn from it. It would be conceivable that this factor could influence the decision to perform or not to perform shoulder surgery in cases where the indication is ambiguous because no clear structural lesion can be evidenced in MR images, even if the patient complains of biceps-related symptoms.

In addition, in patients who are to undergo shoulder surgery due to an existing pathology, such as a rotator cuff lesion, the likelihood of a necessary tenotomy or tenodesis of the long head of the biceps tendon could be better assessed preoperatively if the ratio suggests a pathologically altered LHBT.

4.3. Limitations

The present study is subject to several limitations that must be considered when evaluating the study results. First, this study is subject to a potential selection bias, since only patients with anterior shoulder pain were included in the analysis, and this study is, therefore, missing a control group without LHB tendon pathology. By adding a control group we could have investigated the differences between patients with anterior shoulder pain and healthy asymptomatic individuals. Nevertheless, the aim of the study was to investigate whether the tendon-to-groove ratio can be collected as a reliable parameter and whether the tendon-to-groove ratio can be helpful as a predictive factor for structural

LHB tendon disorders in a tendinopathy cohort with suspected pulley or SLAP lesions but without clear MR graphic evidence.

Secondly, concerning radiographic imaging, only non-contrast MRI and no MR arthrography examinations were included, limiting sensitivity for the detection of SLAP lesions in preoperative scans, potentially impacting the accuracy of the findings. Nevertheless, all patients underwent arthroscopy of the shoulder, which can be considered the diagnostic gold standard for the detection of SLAP lesions and pulley lesions, and the diagnosis of SLAP lesions or pulley lesions was derived solely from the subsequent diagnostic arthroscopy. Therefore, the diagnostic accuracy of the diagnoses within this study can be considered high.

Thirdly, although the interpretation shows a good, or very good, intra- or inter-rater reliability, a certain degree of subjectivity in rating cannot be precluded.

Lastly, since our retrospective study was carried out in a small study population in a preoperativse setting, small differences between the cohorts could have been underestimated. Furthermore, a study population of only 35 patients limits the generalizability of the findings and increases the risk of selection bias. As the predictive value of the LHB/ITG ratio remained uncertain in the present possibly underpowered study, larger studies including a control cohort of asymptomatic patients without LHB tendon disorders have to clarify whether this extended preoperative analysis using the size ratio of the LHB tendon and intertubercular groove has an impact on the predisposition to LHB tendon pathologies.

5. Conclusions

In the pathogenesis of LHB tendon instability, a shallow morphology of the intertubercular groove has been identified as a potential predisposing factor. However, this study is the first to also consider the dimensions of the LHB tendon as a potential influencing factor and introduce the tendon-to-groove ratio of cross-sectional areas as a novel parameter in describing individual local anatomy. While this new parameter demonstrated high inter-rater reliability in this study, no significant differences were observed that could suggest the presence of LHB instability. However, this study was conducted on a cohort of patients with LHB-related anterior shoulder pain, which limits the generalizability of the findings and introduces potential selection bias. Given that this study primarily aimed to introduce the new parameter and demonstrate its reproducible assessment in a relatively small cohort without a healthy control group, further prospective investigations involving a larger study population and a healthy asymptomatic control group are necessary to explore the influence of the size ratio on the pathogenesis of LHB tendon instability and its clinical utility as a predictive factor in targeted preoperative MRI diagnostics. If subsequent studies establish a correlation between the LHB/ITG ratio and a higher likelihood of LHB tendon instability or lesions, preoperative MRI analysis of the LHB and ITG could serve as a diagnostic tool for guiding treatment decisions or predicting outcomes.

Author Contributions: Conceptualization, C.P. and M.K.; methodology, L.H. (Leopold Henssler) and L.H. (Laura Hechinger); validation, J.S., L.K., and L.H. (Leopold Henssler); formal analysis, L.H. (Leopold Henssler) and K.G.; investigation, L.K., J.S., L.H. (Leopold Henssler), and L.H. (Laura Hechinger); resources, K.G.; data curation, L.H. (Leopold Henssler) and M.R.; writing—original draft preparation, L.H. (Leopold Henssler) and K.G.; writing—review and editing, L.K., M.R., K.G., and L.H. (Leopold Henssler); visualization, L.H. (Leopold Henssler) and M.R.; supervision, M.K., V.A., and C.P.; project administration, V.A. All authors have read and agreed to the published version of the manuscript.

Funding: This research received no external funding.

Institutional Review Board Statement: This study was conducted in accordance with the Declaration of Helsinki and approved by the Ethics Committee of the University of Regensburg (protocol number: 18-1032-101).

Informed Consent Statement: Not applicable.

Data Availability Statement: The raw data supporting the conclusions of this article will be made available by the authors on reasonable request.

Conflicts of Interest: The authors declare no conflicts of interest.

References

1. Nho, S.J.; Strauss, E.J.; Lenart, B.A.; Provencher, M.T.; Mazzocca, A.D.; Verma, N.N.; Romeo, A.A. Long head of the biceps tendinopathy: Diagnosis and management. *J. Am. Acad. Orthop. Surg.* **2010**, *18*, 645–656. [CrossRef] [PubMed]
2. Chen, C.H.; Hsu, K.Y.; Chen, W.J.; Shih, C.H. Incidence and Severity of Biceps Long-Head Tendon Lesion in Patients with Complete Rotator Cuff Tears. *J. Trauma.* **2005**, *58*, 1189–1193. [CrossRef] [PubMed]
3. Ahrens, P.M.; Boileau, P. The long head of biceps and associated tendinopathy. *J. Bone Jt. Surg. Br.* **2007**, *89*, 1001–1009. [CrossRef] [PubMed]
4. Saltzman, B.M.; Leroux, T.S.; Cotter, E.J.; Basques, B.; Griffin, J.; Frank, R.M.; Romeo, A.A.; Verma, N.N. Trends in Open and Arthroscopic Long Head of Biceps Tenodesis. *HSS J.* **2020**, *16*, 2–8. [CrossRef]
5. Van Deurzen, D.F.P.; Garssen, F.L.; Kerkhoffs, G.M.M.J.; Bleys, R.L.A.W.; Ten Have, I.; van den Bekerom, M.P.J. Clinical relevance of the anatomy of the long head bicipital groove, an evidence-based review. *Clin. Anat.* **2021**, *34*, 199–208. [CrossRef] [PubMed]
6. Varacallo, M.; Seaman, T.J.; Mair, S.D. *Biceps Tendon Dislocation and Instability*; StatPearls Publishing: Treasure Island, FL, USA, 2023.
7. Lafosse, L.; Reiland, Y.; Baier, G.P.; Toussaint, B.; Jost, B. Anterior and posterior instability of the long head of the biceps tendon in rotator cuff tears: A new classification based on arthroscopic observations. *Arthroscopy* **2007**, *23*, 73–80. [CrossRef] [PubMed]
8. Diplock, B.; Hing, W.; Marks, D. The long head of biceps at the shoulder: A scoping review. *BMC Musculoskelet. Disord.* **2023**, *24*, 232. [CrossRef] [PubMed]
9. Boileau, P.; Ahrens, P.M.; Hatzidakis, A.M. Entrapment of the long head of the biceps tendon: The hourglass biceps—a cause of pain and locking of the shoulder. *J. Shoulder Elb. Surg.* **2004**, *13*, 249–257. [CrossRef] [PubMed]
10. Walch, G.; Nové-Josserand, L.; Boileau, P.; Levigne, C. Subluxations and dislocations of the tendon of the long head of the biceps. *J. Shoulder Elb. Surg.* **1998**, *7*, 100–108. [CrossRef]
11. Martetschläger, F.; Zampeli, F.; Tauber, M.; Habermeyer, P. Lesions of the biceps pulley: A prospective study and classification update. *JSES Int.* **2020**, *4*, 318–323. [CrossRef]
12. Petchprapa, C.N.; Beltran, L.S.; Jazrawi, L.M.; Kwon, Y.W.; Babb, J.S.; Recht, M.P. The rotator interval: A review of anatomy, function, and normal and abnormal MRI appearance. *AJR Am. J. Roentgenol.* **2010**, *195*, 567–576. [CrossRef]
13. Habermeyer, P.; Magosch, P.; Pritsch, M.; Scheibel, M.T.; Lichtenberg, S. Anterosuperior impingement of the shoulder as a result of pulley lesions: A prospective arthroscopic study. *J. Shoulder Elbow Surg.* **2004**, *13*, 5–12. [CrossRef] [PubMed]
14. Hawi, N.; Liodakis, E.; Garving, C.; Habermeyer, P.; Tauber, M. Pulley lesions in rotator cuff tears: Prevalence, etiology, and concomitant pathologies. *Arch. Orthop. Trauma. Surg.* **2017**, *137*, 1097–1105. [CrossRef] [PubMed]
15. Lee, H.I.; Shon, M.S.; Koh, K.H.; Lim, T.K.; Heo, J.; Yoo, J.C. Clinical and radiologic results of arthroscopic biceps tenodesis with suture anchor in the setting of rotator cuff tear. *J. Shoulder Elb. Surg.* **2014**, *23*, e53–e60. [CrossRef] [PubMed]
16. Fischetti, M.; Stoppino, L.P.; Petrera, M.R.; Francavilla, A.; Vinci, R.; Zappia, M.; Macarini, L. MRI morphological evaluation of humeral head bone profile inside region of the biceps pulley reflection. *Skeletal Radiol.* **2022**, *51*, 2017–2025. [CrossRef] [PubMed]
17. Braun, S.; Millett, P.J.; Yongpravat, C.; Pault, J.D.; Anstett, T.; Torry, M.R.; Giphart, J.E. Biomechanical evaluation of shear force vectors leading to injury of the biceps reflection pulley: A biplane fluoroscopy study on cadaveric shoulders. *Am. J. Sports Med.* **2010**, *38*, 1015–1024. [CrossRef] [PubMed]
18. Buck, F.M.; Dietrich, T.J.; Resnick, D.; Jost, B.; Pfirrmann, C.W. Long biceps tendon: Normal position, shape, and orientation in its groove in neutral position and external and internal rotation. *Radiology* **2011**, *261*, 872–881. [CrossRef] [PubMed]
19. Genovese, E.; Spanò, E.; Castagna, A.; Leonardi, A.; Angeretti, M.G.; Callegari, L.; Fugazzola, C. MR-arthrography in superior instability of the shoulder: Correlation with arthroscopy. *Radiol. Med.* **2013**, *118*, 1022–1033. [CrossRef]
20. Kim, J.Y.; Rhee, S.M.; Rhee, Y.G. Accuracy of MRI in diagnosing intra-articular pathology of the long head of the biceps tendon: Results with a large cohort of patients. *BMC Musculoskelet. Disord.* **2019**, *20*, 270. [CrossRef]
21. Abboud, J.A.; Bartolozzi, A.R.; Widmer, B.J.; DeMola, P.M. Bicipital groove morphology on MRI has no correlation to intra-articular biceps tendon pathology. *J. Shoulder Elb. Surg.* **2010**, *19*, 790–794. [CrossRef]
22. Pfahler, M.; Branner, S.; Refior, H.J. The role of the bicipital groove in tendopathy of the long biceps tendon. *J. Shoulder Elb. Surg.* **1999**, *8*, 419–424. [CrossRef] [PubMed]
23. Shah, S.H.; Small, K.M.; Sinz, N.J.; Higgins, L.D. Morphology of the Lesser Tuberosity and Intertubercular Groove in Patients with Arthroscopically Confirmed Subscapularis and Biceps Tendon Pathology. *Arthroscopy* **2016**, *32*, 968–975. [CrossRef] [PubMed]
24. Kavak, R.P.; Ozdemir, M.; Duman, E. Effects of bicipital groove bony morphology on the stability of long head of the biceps tendon. *Eurasian J. Med.* **2019**, *3*, 293–299. [CrossRef]
25. Ulucakoy, C.; Kaptan, A.Y.; Yapar, A.; Orhan, O.; Ozer, M.; Kanatli, U. The effect of bicipital groove morphology on the stability of the biceps long head tendon. *Arch. Orthop. Trauma. Surg.* **2021**, *141*, 1325–1330. [CrossRef] [PubMed]
26. Yoo, J.C.; Iyyampillai, G.; Park, D.; Koh, K.H. The influence of bicipital groove morphology on the stability of the long head of the biceps tendon. *J Orthop. Surg.* **2017**, *25*, 2309499017717195. [CrossRef] [PubMed]

27. Spritzer, C.E.; Collins, A.J.; Cooperman, A.; Speer, K.P. Assessment of instability of the long head of the biceps tendon by MRI. *Skelet. Radiol.* **2001**, *30*, 199–207. [CrossRef] [PubMed]
28. Kleim, B.D.; Carbonel, J.F.S.; Hinz, M.; Rupp, M.C.; Scheiderer, B.; Imhoff, A.B.; Siebenlist, S. A shallow morphology of the intertubercular groove is associated with medial and bilateral but not lateral pulley lesions. *Knee Surg. Sports Traumatol. Arthrosc.* **2023**, *31*, 3221–3229. [CrossRef]
29. Cardoso, A.; Freire, G.; Alonso, R.; Afonso, P.D.; Pires, L. Bicipital groove cross-sectional area on ultrasonography: Does a correlation to intra-articular tendon pathology exist? *Orthop. Traumatol. Surg. Res.* **2021**, *107*, 102747. [CrossRef]

Journal of
Clinical Medicine

MDPI

Article

Clinical and Surgical Outcomes of Shoulder Arthrodesis

Salar Sobhi [1,*], Kieran Bochat [1,2], Grant Booth [2], Andrew Mattin [1] and Sheldon Moniz [1]

[1] Department of Orthopaedic Surgery, The Orthopaedic Research Foundation of Western Australia (ORFWA), Murdoch, WA 6150, Australia
[2] Department of Orthopaedic Surgery, Royal Perth Hospital, Perth, WA 6000, Australia
* Correspondence: salar.sobhi@health.wa.gov.au; Tel.: +61-403461850

Abstract: Introduction: Shoulder arthrodesis is typically seen as a salvage procedure with limited functional objectives. In appropriately selected patients, it may effectively alleviate pain, provide stable motion, and offer patient function satisfaction. However, there have been few reports on the outcomes following shoulder arthrodesis. **Methods:** A multicenter, retrospective chart review of patients undergoing shoulder arthrodesis between 2001 and 2023 in Western Australia was conducted. Clinical records and imaging were then reviewed to determine patient demographics. A cross-sectional analysis of Visual Analogue (VAS), Oxford Shoulder (OSS), and American Shoulder and Elbow Surgeons Shoulder (ASES) Scores, satisfaction and complication rates was conducted. **Results:** In total, 14 patients with a mean age of 39.5 years (range 22–52 years, 71% male) with a mean follow-up of 7.4 years (range 3 months 18 years) were identified. The most common indications for arthrodesis included osteoarthritis (8, 57%) and instability (6, 43%). Major contributory factors were recurrent seizures (5, 36%) and multiple surgeries (4, 29%). Radiographic union was observed in 13 (93%) patients. The mean VAS was 2.8 (range 0–7), mean OSS was 33.0 (range 23–42) and ASES score was 55.4 (range 37–82). In total, 11 patients (79%) reported being satisfied. Five (36%) patients returned to theatre for complications. **Conclusions**: In this patient series, shoulder arthrodesis demonstrates a notable efficacy in pain reduction, high satisfaction, acceptable function, and complication rates.

Keywords: shoulder arthrodesis; glenohumeral joint arthrodesis

1. Introduction

Shoulder joint arthrodesis is generally considered a salvage procedure that aims to provide a painless and stable shoulder position to allow function using scapulothoracic, elbow, and hand motion [1]. Shoulder arthrodesis has been employed less in recent years with improved techniques and prostheses relating to reverse shoulder arthroplasty. Common indications for shoulder arthrodesis include brachial plexopathies, refractory instability, significant glenohumeral bone loss, deltoid and rotator cuff deficiency, and chronic infections [2,3]. The rotator cuff muscles work not only as a motion actuator (abduction or external and internal rotations) but also as a shoulder stabilizer. In the case of untreated rotator cuff tears, the humeral head can move upward and rub against the acromion, resulting in glenohumeral joint arthropathy.

Shoulder arthrodesis can be achieved using intra-articular and extra-articular techniques [1]. Most commonly, compression screws or plate fixation are employed for this procedure [4–6]. Despite the unique set of indications and goals of this procedure, shoulder arthrodesis is not commonly performed as revision shoulder arthroplasty has equivalent relief rates and improved functional outcomes. Shoulder arthrodesis can still be an option for patients who have undergone multiple failed revision arthroplasties or those with glenohumeral arthritis accompanied by rotator cuff and deltoid muscle dysfunction, as it may offer a more predictable outcome [7].

Despite improvements in modern materials and techniques, shoulder arthrodesis is associated with complication rates as high as 43% [1,8,9]. These include but are not limited to component malposition, infection and non-union. Outcomes following shoulder arthrodesis are seldom reported in the literature. This is due to the heterogeneity of patient indications, variations in techniques and arthrodesis methods, and lack of long-term follow-up. Few studies exist investigating shoulder arthrodesis in a larger cohort of mixed indications, and many of these do not report outcomes using standardised function scores [1].

This retrospective review aims to report the subjective and objective short- and long-term results of shoulder arthrodesis for 14 patients.

2. Methods

2.1. Patients

This was a multi-centre, multi-surgeon retrospective review of patients who underwent shoulder arthrodesis between 2001 and 2023 in Western Australia. The procedures were performed in three high-volume tertiary orthopaedic centres by four orthopaedic surgeons with a subspecialty interest in shoulder surgery.

Inclusion criteria—patients who underwent shoulder arthrodesis during the aforementioned time period and were above 18 years of age at the time of data collection for this study.

Exclusion criteria—patients with mental compromise (i.e., currently being treated for a psychiatric disorder, senile dementia, Alzheimer's disease, presence of alcohol and/or substance abuse), or an inability to provide informed consent.

This study was conducted according to the guidelines of the Declaration of Helsinki and approved by the South Metropolitan Health Service Governance Evidence Knowledge Outcomes (GEKO) Committee (GEKO approval No. 42649). All participants provided informed consent for data collection for this study.

2.2. Operative Technique and Rehabilitation

All patients underwent a general anaesthetic, were in a supine position with a beach chair, and received perioperative antibiotics. An S-shaped skin incision beginning over the scapular spine, traversing anteriorly over the acromion, and extending down the anterolateral aspect of the arm was employed in all cases. The patient's passive ability to move their hand to their mouth and face intra-operatively was used as the arthrodesis position, which was generally 30° abduction, 30° internal rotation, and 30° forward flexion. Plate and screw constructs were used in all cases (Figure 1).

All patients underwent post-operative multimodal analgesia and input from the hospital's acute pain service. All patients underwent sling immobilisation for at least 6 weeks post-operatively. All patients underwent serial clinical and radiological review post-operatively to assess efficacy of the arthrodesis (Figure 1).

2.3. Baseline Demographics

A retrospective review of patient's medical records was conducted. Baseline demographics including age, sex, hand dominance, side of surgery, occupation, date of surgery, and indications for arthrodesis, past medical history including smoking status, drug and opioid use were collected.

2.4. Assessment of Clinical Outcomes

In this cross-sectional study, patients were interviewed and had their clinical outcomes assessed using the Visual Analogue Scale (VAS), Oxford Shoulder Score (OSS), and American Shoulder and Elbow Surgeons Standardised Shoulder (ASES) scores. Patient were also asked if they were satisfied with their arthrodesis.

Visual Analogue Scale (VAS)—A validated, subjective measure for acute and chronic pain. Patient scores were recorded by making a handwritten mark on a 10 cm line that represents a continuum between "no pain" and "worst pain" [10].

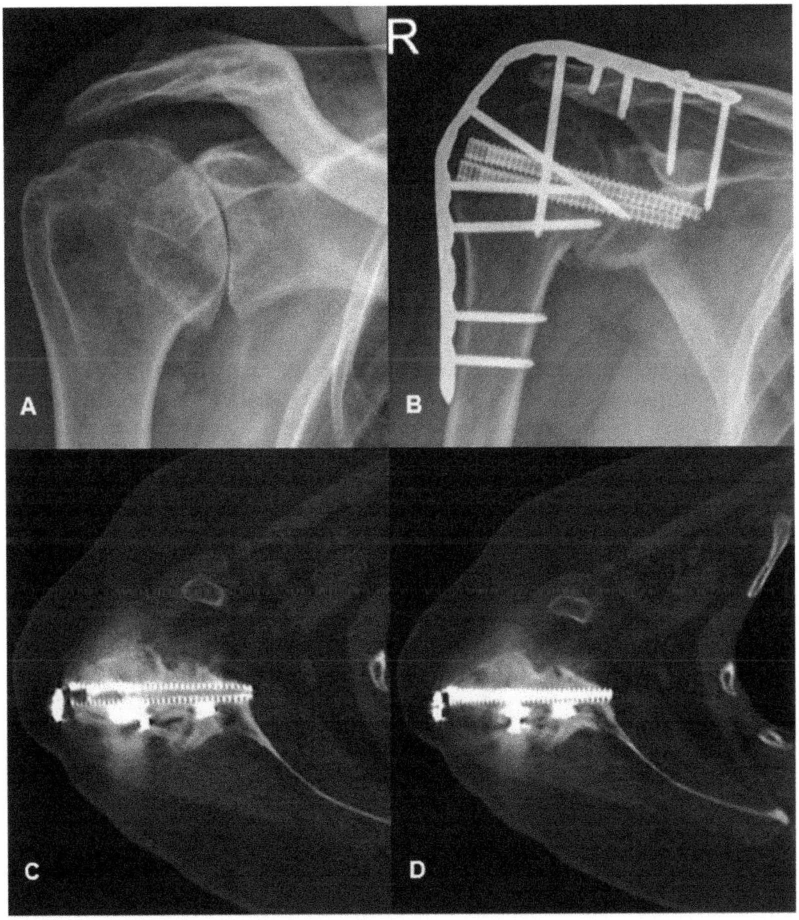

Figure 1. (**A**) shows an anteroposterior radiograph of the right shoulder demonstrating evidence of osteoarthritis in a patient with recurrent septic arthritis. (**B**) shows the same patient undergoing shoulder arthrodesis with screw and plate constructs. (**C**,**D**) are post-operative axial computed tomography scans demonstrating bridging callus and arthrodesis of the shoulder joint.

Oxford Shoulder Score (OSS)—A validated scoring system used to assess the degree of pain and disability caused by shoulder pathology [11]. It contains 12 items, each with 5 potential answers. A mark between 1 (best/fewest symptoms) and 5 (worst/most severe) is awarded to correspond to the patient's symptoms. The combined total gives a minimum score of 12 and a maximum of 60. A higher score implies a greater degree of disability [12].

American Shoulder and Elbow Surgeons Standardised Shoulder (ASES) Score—A validated joint-specific score used to assess shoulder pain and function. The ASES is a 100-point scale that assess the following three sections: pain, instability, and activities of daily living. The combined total gives a minimum score of 0 and a maximum of 100, of which 50 is attributed to pain. A high score implied a greater degree of function, stability, and less pain [13].

Additionally, complications that required patients to return to the operating room were noted and analysed.

2.5. Statistical Analyses

Given the cross-sectional nature of this study, proportions were presented as percentages (%). Averages of functional outcomes VAS, OSS and ASES were presented as means and range.

3. Results

3.1. Patient Characteristics

Table 1 shows the demographic data, complications, and functional results of all patients. A total of 14 patients with a mean age of 39.5 years (range 22–52 years) with a mean follow-up of 7.4 years (range 3 months–18 years) were identified in our multi-hospital database. Most cases (10 out of 14, 71%) undergoing shoulder arthrodesis were male, involved their dominant limb (9 out of 14, 64%), and were unemployed (8 out of 14, 57%). Furthermore, 4 (29%) patients experienced opioid dependence and 8 (57%) were active smokers at the time of review.

The most common indication for shoulder arthrodesis was osteoarthritis (8 out of 14, 57%), followed by instability (6 out of 14, 43%). The major contributory factors for performing shoulder arthrodesis were recurrent seizures (5 out of 14, 36%) and multiple failed surgeries (4 out of 14, 29%). A total of 4 out of 14 patients (29%) in this cohort had a previous or current history of intravenous drug use (IVDU).

3.2. Outcomes

Out of the 14 patients, 13 (93%) achieved radiographic union. The mean pain score measured through the VAS was 2.8 (range 0–7). The mean OSS of the cohort was 33.0 (range 23–42). The mean ASES score was 55.4 (range 37–82). A total of 11 out of 14 patients (79%) reported being satisfied with their procedure at the time of reporting.

3.3. Complications

A total of five (36%) patients returned to the operating room for complications. One patient required revision arthrodesis due to malunion. Two required metalwork removal for infection and one for prominent metalwork. One patient who underwent shoulder arthrodesis for osteoarthritis secondary to recurrent seizures underwent conversion to reverse total shoulder replacement due to ongoing pain and lack of callus formation at four months post-arthrodesis (Figure 2). Lastly, one patient is awaiting elective plate removal.

Table 1. Outcomes of patients following shoulder arthrodesis.

A	B	C	D	E	F	G	H	I	J	K	L	M	N
35	F	N	Y	N	N	Humeral head AVN Axillary nerve palsy	Multiple surgeries	18	3	38	40	Nil	Y
35	M	N	N	Y	N	Humeral head AVN	Multiple surgeries	7	7	41	30	Nil	N
38	M	Y	N	N	Y	GHJ OA Rotator cuff insufficiency	IVDU	5	2	68	36	Malunion, required revision	Y
45	M	N	N	N	N	GHJ OA Axillary nerve palsy Instability	Seizures	5	2	45	41	Washout, plate removal for infection	Y
27	M	Y	Y	Y	Y	GHJ OA Instability	Multiple surgeries	4	2	62	38	Removal of plate due to irritation, CRPS	Y
33	M	Y	Y	N	N	Erb's palsy GHJ OA		8	0	56	23	Nil	Y
22	F	Y	Y	N	N	Chronic anterior dislocation	Seizures	7	4	42	33	Nil	Y
42	M	N	N	N	Y	Instability	Seizures, IVDU, TBI	11	0	82	26	Nil	Y
48	M	Y	Y	N	Y	GHJ OA	IVDU	10	0	70	23	Nil	Y
43	M	Y	Y	N	Y	GHJ OA Instability		8	4	58	27	Nil	Y
50	F	Y	N	Y	Y	GHJ OA	RA, previous SA	9	4	56	32	Infection, removal of metalwork	Y
47	M	Y	N	Y	Y	Humeral head AVN	IVDU, schizophrenia	10	0	48	29	Planned plate removal	N
36	F	N	N	N	N	Instability	Seizures Multiple surgeries	9 m	4	73	42	Nil	Y
52	M	Y	N	N	Y	GHJ OA	Seizures	4 m	7	37	42	Lack of callus. Converted to rTSR.	N

A—age at operation; B—sex; C—dominant limb; D—employed; E—opioid dependence; F—smoker; G—indication; H—contributory factors; I—follow-up (years); J—visual analogue score; K—ASES score; L—Oxford shoulder score; M—complications; N—satisfied.

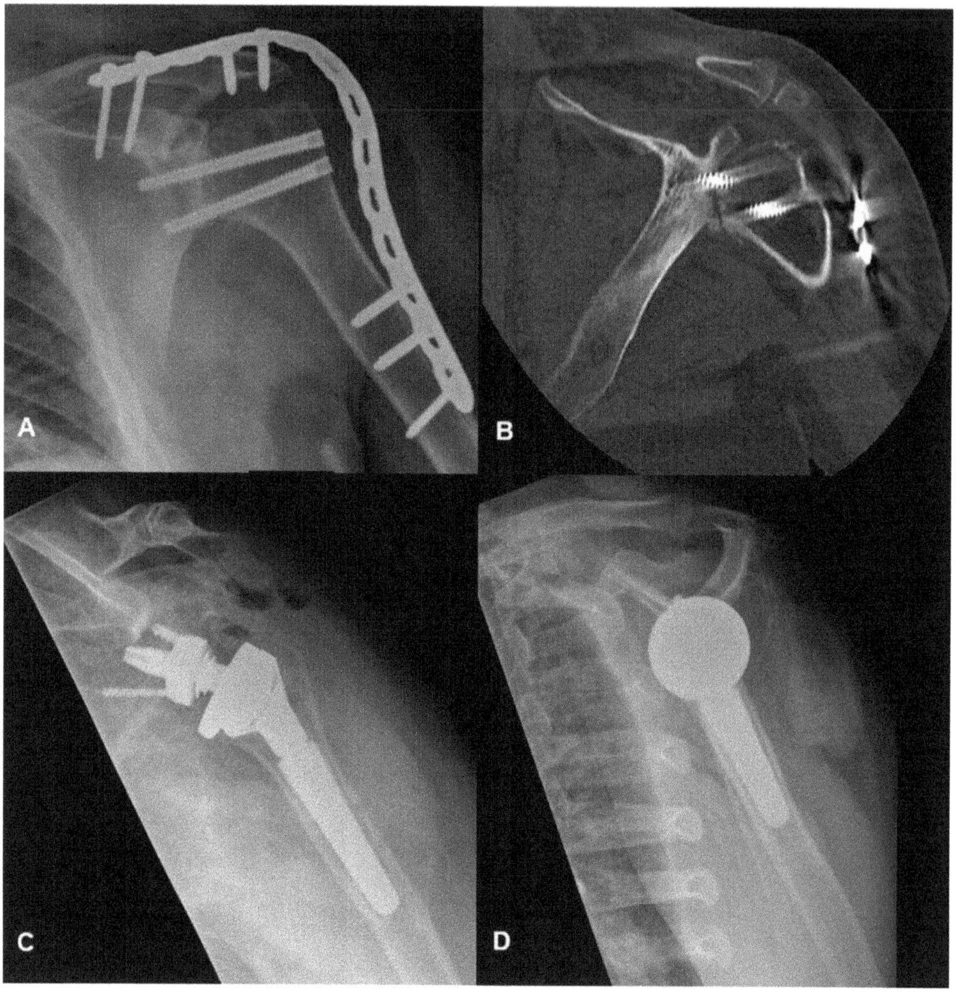

Figure 2. (**A**) shows an anteroposterior radiograph of the left shoulder of a patient with ongoing pain and mobility 4 months post-shoulder arthrodesis for osteoarthritis and recurrent seizures. (**B**) shows a post-operative axial computed tomography scan demonstrating lack of bridging callus formation. (**C**,**D**) are post-operative radiographs of the same patient undergoing reverse total shoulder arthroplasty after being seizure-free for 12 months.

4. Discussion

To date, our cross-sectional study is one of the largest to contribute to the small body of literature available relating to outcomes following shoulder arthrodesis with plate and screw fixation. In this cohort, shoulder arthrodesis was predominantly performed in young males with osteoarthritis or instability. Major contributory factors to having this procedure included recurrent seizures, multiple surgeries, and history of IVDU. Our results showed acceptable functional scores, high union (93%), and satisfaction rates (79%). The post-operative complication rate requiring return to the operating room for this procedure was 36%.

The indication for shoulder arthrodesis has decreased in the last few years due to recent advances in surgical techniques and arthroplasty. However, it is still considered a salvage procedure in specific patients with paralytic or pseudoparalytic shoulders, chronic refractory instability, infection, failed arthroplasty, or after tumour resection [14]. Despite the limited function achieved with this procedure, it improves pain and patients were generally satisfied in the context of their significant co-morbidities in this patient series.

4.1. Outcomes

The objective outcomes of shoulder arthrodesis in our cohort demonstrated acceptable scores comparable to those undergoing shoulder arthroplasty and previous arthrodesis cohorts in the literature. Given the inability for shoulder arthrodesis patients to elevate their arm to 90°, only the VAS, OSS and ASES shoulder index were employed in this study. The mean OSS of 33.0 (range 23–42) found in our cohort is considered an acceptable result when compared with patients undergoing shoulder arthroplasty, where a patient-acceptable symptom state (PASS) has been defined as a score above 29 Similarly [15], our mean VAS of 2.8 (range 0–7) and ASES of 55.4 (range 37–82) were similar to Dimmen et al.'s (2007) cohort of 18 shoulder arthrodesis patients who were followed-up between 3 and 15 years who and who had mean VAS and ASES scores of 1.6 (range 0–8) and 59 (15–95), respectively[4] Conversely, the mean ASES score of our cohort was significantly lower than the acceptable PASS estimate of 76 for patients undergoing shoulder arthroplasty [16]. This can be explained as the ASES has many components that assess the ability to perform overhead activities that are not possible following arthrodesis, thus resulting in lower scores. Additionally, it is known that shoulder arthroplasty results in a superior range of motion and therefore function.

4.2. Satisfaction

Similarly, our high satisfaction rate of 79% is consistent with previously published literature. Górecki et al.'s (2021) systematic review of 294 patients undergoing shoulder arthrodesis for brachial plexus injury reported a subjective satisfaction rate of 82% (range 59–100%) and similarly, Dimmen et al.'s (2007) cohort reported a satisfaction rate of 83% relative to their pre-operative condition [4,8]. Furthermore, there is no difference in satisfaction when comparing plate and screw stabilisation in the literature [8]. Given the chronic pain, instability and multiple surgeries seen in this cohort, a definitive procedure to help address these issues allowing an acceptable level of pain and function, with the ability to perform basic everyday activities such as eating or personal hygiene, may attribute to this high satisfaction rate.

4.3. Complications

Our reported complication rate requiring return to the operating room was 36%. Additionally, another two patients in the cohort had planned metalwork removal. Recent studies show that the incidence of all complications following shoulder arthrodesis is 28%, and has been reported as high as 43% [8].Early complications are infrequent and include surgical site infection, breakdown of skin and haematoma formation[8] Later complications include non-union, being as high as 20% in some series, infection, malunion, periprosthetic fracture, hardware prominence and irritation.

Ruhmann et al. (2002) showed that 9% of patients had non-union [17]. This was followed by another series in 2005 that showed that the union rate was high in plate compared to screw arthrodesis [18]. Dimmen et al. (2007) demonstrated a union rate of 89% with 2 out of 18 patients demonstrating asymptomatic partial fusion (glenohumeral or acromiohumeral) radiographically [4]. This was similar to our radiographic union rate of 93%, with our single case of non-union converted to a reverse total shoulder arthroplasty at 4 months post-arthrodesis.

The infection rate following shoulder arthrodesis is reported to range between 0 and 14%. In our cohort, where all patients received perioperative antibiotics, we demonstrated a 14% infection rate (2 out of 14 patients), requiring removal of metalwork and washout. Furthermore, periprosthetic fracture rates following shoulder arthrodesis are reported to be up to 11% in the literature. A combination of an immobile shoulder joint, osteopenia and development of a stress riser due to the plate can result in periprosthetic fracture. Cofield and Briggs (1979) had eight fractures in their series of 71 patients (11%), whilst no fractures were reported in our cohort or in Richards et al. (1988) and Stark et al.'s (1991) cohorts [2,5,6]. Lastly, we had one case of plate removal due to irritation and one planned elective plate removal. Several studies have demonstrated the need for hardware removal after union for symptomatic plates and/or screws [5,6,9]. Most commonly, irritation occurs over the scapular spine and acromion due to less soft tissue coverage [9].

4.4. Limitations

This study must be viewed considering its limitations. Firstly, data collection was retrospective and functional outcomes were obtained cross-sectionally. Therefore, we are unable to ascertain the outcomes of shoulder arthrodesis over time. Secondly, the single-arm nature of this study makes interpretation of outcomes difficult, given there is no cohort for comparison. Thirdly, we were unable to collect data on certain outcomes such as range of motion, which makes it difficult to ascertain what level of function is possible in our cohort. Lastly, the wide range of follow-up (3 months to 18 years) makes it difficult to accurately quote a complication rate; however, it is historically known that shoulder arthrodesis has frequent complications.

5. Conclusions

In our cross-sectional review of 14 patients identified as suitable candidates for salvage procedures addressing diverse shoulder pathologies, shoulder arthrodesis demonstrated notable efficacy in pain reduction. Furthermore, it has the potential to attain a satisfactory level of function and subjective contentment in the best-case scenario.

Author Contributions: Conceptualization, A.M. and G.B.; methodology, K.B.; software, S.M.; validation, A.M., G.B. and S.M.; formal analysis, S.S.; investigation, S.S.; resources, S.M.; data curation, S.S.; writing—original draft preparation, S.S.; writing—review and editing, S.M.; visualization, K.B.; supervision, A.M.; project administration, A.M. All authors have read and agreed to the published version of the manuscript.

Funding: There is no external funding source.

Institutional Review Board Statement: The study was conducted in accordance with the Declaration of Helsinki, and approved by the Institutional Review Board (or Ethics Committee) of Fiona Stanley and Fremantle Hospital Group (Governance Evidence Knowledge Outcome Code 12496, approval date is 23 December 2023).

Informed Consent Statement: Informed consent was obtained from all subjects involved in the study.

Data Availability Statement: The data presented in this study are available on request from the corresponding author.

Conflicts of Interest: The authors declare no conflict of interest.

References

1. Del Core, M.A.; Cutler, H.S.; Schacherer, T.; Khazzam, M. Glenohumeral arthrodesis. *JSES Rev. Rep. Tech.* **2021**, *1*, 367–372. [CrossRef] [PubMed]
2. Cofield, R.H.; Briggs, B. Glenohumeral arthrodesis. Operative and long-term functional results. *JBJS* **1979**, *61*, 668–677. [CrossRef]
3. Charnley, J. Compression arthrodesis of the ankle and shoulder. *J. Bone Jt. Surg.* **1951**, *33*, 180–191. [CrossRef]
4. Dimmen, S.; Madsen, J.E. Long-term outcome of shoulder arthrodesis performed with plate fixation: 18 patients examined after 3–15 years. *Acta Orthop.* **2007**, *78*, 827–833. [CrossRef] [PubMed]
5. Stark, D.M.; Bennett, J.B.; Tullos, H.S. *Rigid Internal Fixation for Shoulder Arthrodesis*; SLACK Incorporated: Thorofare, NJ, USA, 1991; Volume 14, pp. 849–855.
6. Richards, R.R.; Sherman, R.; Hudson, A.; Waddell, J. Shoulder arthrodesis using a pelvic-reconstruction plate. A report of eleven cases. *JBJS* **1988**, *70*, 416–421. [CrossRef]
7. Wagner, E.R.; McLaughlin, R.; Sarfani, S.; Cofield, R.H.; Sperling, J.W.; Sanchez-Sotelo, J.; Elhassan, B.T. Long-term outcomes of glenohumeral arthrodesis. *JBJS* **2018**, *100*, 598–604. [CrossRef] [PubMed]

8. Górecki, M.; Czarnecki, P. The influence of shoulder arthrodesis on the function of the upper limb in adult patients after a brachial plexus injury: A systematic literature review with elements of meta-analysis. *EFORT Open Rev.* **2021**, *6*, 797–807. [CrossRef] [PubMed]
9. Kamineni, S.; Unger, R.Z.; Desai, R. Shoulder arthrodesis in the management of glenohumeral pathologies. *J. Shoulder Elb. Arthroplast.* **2019**, *3*, 2471549219850655. [CrossRef]
10. Carlsson, A.M. Assessment of chronic pain. I. Aspects of the reliability and validity of the visual analogue scale. *Pain* **1983**, *16*, 87–101. [CrossRef] [PubMed]
11. Angst, F.; Schwyzer, H.K.; Aeschlimann, A.; Simmen, B.R.; Goldhahn, J. Measures of adult shoulder function: Disabilities of the arm, shoulder, and hand questionnaire (DASH) and its short version (QuickDASH), shoulder pain and disability index (SPADI), American shoulder and elbow surgeons (ASES) society standardized shoulder assessment form, constant (Murley) score (CS), simple shoulder test (SST), oxford shoulder score (OSS), shoulder disability questionnaire (SDQ), and Western Ontario shoulder instability index (WOSI). *Arthritis Care Res.* **2011**, *63*, S174–S188.
12. Dawson, J.; Fitzpatrick, R. Questionnaire on the perceptions of patients about shoulder surgery. *J. Bone Jt. Surg.* **1996**, *78*, 593–600. [CrossRef]
13. Kocher, M.S.; Horan, M.P.; Briggs, K.K.; Richardson, T.R.; O'Holleran, J.; Hawkins, R.J. Reliability, validity, and responsiveness of the American Shoulder and Elbow Surgeons subjective shoulder scale in patients with shoulder instability, rotator cuff disease, and glenohumeral arthritis. *JBJS* **2005**, *87*, 2006–2011. [CrossRef]
14. Safran, O.; Iannotti, J.P. Arthrodesis of the shoulder. *JAAOS-J. Am. Acad. Orthop. Surg.* **2006**, *14*, 145–153. [CrossRef] [PubMed]
15. Liu, P.; Afzal, I.; Asopa, V.; Clement, N.D.; Patel, V. Changes and thresholds in the Oxford Shoulder Score following shoulder arthroplasty: Minimal clinically important difference, minimal important and detectable changes, and patient-acceptable symptom state. *Shoulder Elb.* **2023**, 17585732231176423. [CrossRef]
16. Chamberlain, A.M.; Hung, M.; Chen, W.; Keener, J.D.; McAllister, J.; Ebersole, G.; Granger, E.K.; Bowen, R.C.; Tashjian, R.Z. Determining the patient acceptable symptomatic state for the ASES, SST, and VAS pain after total shoulder arthroplasty. *J. Shoulder Elb. Arthroplast.* **2017**, *1*, 2471549217720042. [CrossRef]
17. Rühmann, O.; Clare, D.J.; Wirth, M.A.; Groh, G.I.; Rockwood, C.A., Jr. Pseudarthrosis after shoulder arthrodesis. *J. Bone Joint Surg. Am.* **2002**, *84*, 874–876. [CrossRef] [PubMed]
18. Rühmann, O.; Schmolke, S.; Bohnsack, M.; Flamme, C.; Wirth, C.J. Shoulder arthrodesis: Indications, technique, results, and complications. *J. Shoulder Elbow Surg.* **2005**, *14*, 38–50. [CrossRef] [PubMed]

Journal of
Clinical Medicine

MDPI

Article

Clinical and Structural Results Following Arthroscopic and Open Repair of Isolated Subscapularis Tears

Christoph Bartl [1,2,*], Janna Dolde [1], Florian Gebhard [1], Stefan Eichhorn [3], Lisa Hainzer [4] and Stephan Pauly [4,5]

1 Department of Orthopaedic Trauma Surgery, Ulm University, Albert-Einstein-Allee 23, 89081 Ulm, Germany; sekretariat.unfallchirurgie@uniklinik-ulm.de (J.D.); florian.gebhard@uniklinik-ulm.de (F.G.)
2 Center of Orthopaedic and Sports Medicine, Rosa-Bavaresestr. 1, 80639 Munich, Germany
3 Department of Biomechanics, TÜV Süd, Munich Ridlerstr. 65, 80635 Munich, Germany; stefan.eichhorn@tuvsud.com
4 Department of Shoulder and Elbow Surgery, Vivantes Auguste-Viktoria-Klinikum, Rubensstr. 125, 12157 Berlin, Germany; schulter.avk@vivantes.de (L.H.); stephan.pauly@vivantes.de (S.P.)
5 Department of Clinical Medicine, Medical School Berlin, Rüdesheimerstr. 50, 14197 Berlin, Germany
* Correspondence: chbartl@gmx.de

Abstract: Objective: With advances in techniques, arthroscopic repair of isolated subscapularis tendon tears has become increasingly popular in recent years. The aim of this study was to analyze the clinical and structural results of arthroscopic repair versus the gold standard of open repair. It is a prospective cohort study with a control group; evidence level III. **Methods:** In a prospective study performed at two centers, 18 patients with an isolated subscapularis tear were treated with arthroscopic repair (ARG) and 16 patients with open repair (ORG) using a uniform single-row suture anchor repair technique in both groups. The subscapularis function was assessed using specific clinical tests (belly-press and lift-off tests), strength testing and shoulder function with the use of the Constant–Murley score (CMS). Standardized magnetic resonance imaging (MRI) was used to evaluate the postoperative subscapularis muscle-tendon status. **Results:** At a minimum follow-up of 48 months, the CMS increased from a mean of 54 points preoperatively to a mean of 86 points postoperatively in the ARG ($p < 0.01$) and from 50 points to 85 points postoperatively in the ORG ($p < 0.01$). Specific subscapularis tests (belly-press test and lift-off test) were significantly improved from the preoperative to the postoperative status in both repair groups ($p < 0.05$). Despite a subscapularis tendon healing rate of over 90% on MRI scans in both repair groups, the incomplete correction of specific muscle tests was a frequent postoperative finding. **Conclusions:** Arthroscopic repair of isolated subscapularis tears achieved equivalent clinical and structural results compared to the gold standard of open repair.

Keywords: arthroscopic subscapularis repair; open subscapularis repair; subscapularis test; subscapularis muscle atrophy; subscapularis MRI

1. Introduction

Isolated tendon tears of the subscapularis are relatively rare compared to single tendon supraspinatus tears or combined rotator cuff tears and comprise about 4% of all rotator cuff tears [1,2]. Most subscapularis tears are of degenerative origin and part of a massive rotator cuff tear [1,3]. In contrast, isolated subscapularis tears are often of traumatic origin and show a high percentage of concomitant lesions of the long head of the biceps tendon [1,4,5].

The subscapularis musculotendinous unit provides a substantial biomechanical role for the shoulder as the single anterior part of the stabilizing rotator cuff.

It acts as the main internal rotator of the shoulder and is the single anterior stabilizing part of the transversal force couple of the glenohumeral joint [6]. Untreated, chronic subscapularis tears lead to anterior subluxation of the humeral head and joint degeneration; therefore, subscapularis repair is essential to maintain glenohumeral joint biomechanics [7].

Open subscapularis repair was set as the gold standard for the treatment of isolated subscapularis tears over thirty years ago and achieved good-to-excellent clinical and structural results in many studies [1,8,9]. Over the last two decades, arthroscopic rotator cuff repair, especially of superior and posterosuperior tendon tears, along with significant improvements in arthroscopic equipment and fixation techniques, has evolved as the new surgical standard [10,11]. Due to anatomic characteristics with a narrow anterior joint space in the subscapularis region, exaggerated by the increasing swelling during the arthroscopic procedure over time, the transition to an all-arthroscopic subscapularis repair approach was delayed, and open repair still remained the gold standard [12]. With the increasing experience of arthroscopic surgeons at specialized arthroscopy centers, arthroscopic subscapularis repair yielded similar clinical and structural results compared to open repair studies, as shown in outcome studies and three systematic reviews, but still, a comparative study is not available [1,13–16].

The purpose of this comparative study was to evaluate the clinical and structural midterm results following arthroscopic repair compared to the gold standard of open repair for isolated subscapularis tears using a comparable tendon fixation technique. We hypothesized that there would be no significant differences in clinical outcomes and structural integrity between the two groups.

2. Materials and Methods

At two institutions, all patients with an isolated subscapularis tendon tear between 2012 and 2020 were included in our prospective non-randomized study. The intervention was performed by two surgeons at the two centers, both familiar with open and arthroscopic repair techniques (CB and SP). The ethics committee approved the study (university of Ulm; reference 192/14) and written informed consent was obtained from all patients. A total of 18 patients with arthroscopic repair (the arthroscopic repair group—ARG) and 16 patients with open repair (the open repair group—ORG) completed the study and were available for the final follow-up evaluation.

Patients were finally included in the study if an isolated full-thickness subscapularis tendon tear was confirmed at diagnostic arthroscopy. We excluded partial articular-sided subscapularis tears and tears with involvement of the supraspinatus and infraspinatus tendon. All patients underwent subsequent arthroscopic or open tendon repair, applying a uniform single-row suture anchor repair technique at both centers.

Baseline patient characteristics showed a similar distribution in both groups and are listed in Table 1.

Table 1. Preoperative patient demographics.

	Arthroscopic Repair Group	Open Repair Group	p Value
Number of shoulders	18	16	
Mean age, y (range)	51 (28–62)	54 (33–66)	0.52
Gender			
Male/Female	78%/22%	81%/19%	0.81
Duration Symptomatic onset To surgery (months)	5.5 (1–9)	6.8 (0.5–11)	0.16
Traumatic tear (%)	89%	81%	0.87
Dominant side affected (%)	76%	71%	0.61
Tear size Lafosse classification			
Type II	5	4	
Type III	7	6	
Type IV	6	6	

2.1. Clinical Evaluation

Patients were evaluated with the simple shoulder test (SST) and the Constant–Murley score (CMS) preoperatively and postoperatively [17]. Shoulder range of motion, including flexion, abduction and external rotation with the arm at the side, was measured with an electronic goniometer, and internal rotation was evaluated with a hand on the back preoperatively and at follow-up. Specific assessment of the subscapularis was performed with the belly-press test and the lift-off test preoperatively and at follow-up [18]. The belly-press test results were graded as "negative" for a normal test with full ability to maintain internal rotation during the test, "positive" if internal rotation could not be maintained, and "intermediate" if internal rotation could be maintained partially. Manual subscapularis strength testing was performed in the belly-press and lift-off positions in both repair groups at baseline and follow-up, using the standard classification of neurologic assessment with a strength scale from 0 (minimal strength) to 5 (maximal strength).

2.2. Magnetic Resonance Imaging

Preoperative magnetic resonance imaging (MRI) scans were undertaken to evaluate the tear configuration and subscapularis muscle status with muscle atrophy and muscle fatty infiltration. The fatty infiltration grade (FIG) of the subscapularis muscle was graded using the MRI grading system described by Fuchs et al. based on the adapted Goutallier CT score [19]. Fatty infiltration with FIG 0 and FIG 1 was considered minimal fatty infiltration, representing a normal condition of the study population, FIG 2 moderate and FIG 3 and 4 advanced fatty infiltration of the muscle.

On postoperative MRI scans, subscapularis tendon repair integrity was graded on axial T2-weighted images using the Sugaya classification, with types 1, 2 and 3 graded as intact tendons (Figure 1a) and types 4 and 5 with tendon discontinuity graded as a retear [20,21]. Subscapularis muscle atrophy was evaluated on the Y-shaped view in the sagittal plane: no atrophy (grade 0), mild atrophy (grade 1), moderate atrophy (grade 2) and advanced atrophy (grade 3) (Figure 1b,c). The MRI scans were graded separately by two investigators (CB and SP) and in consensus in case of discrepancy.

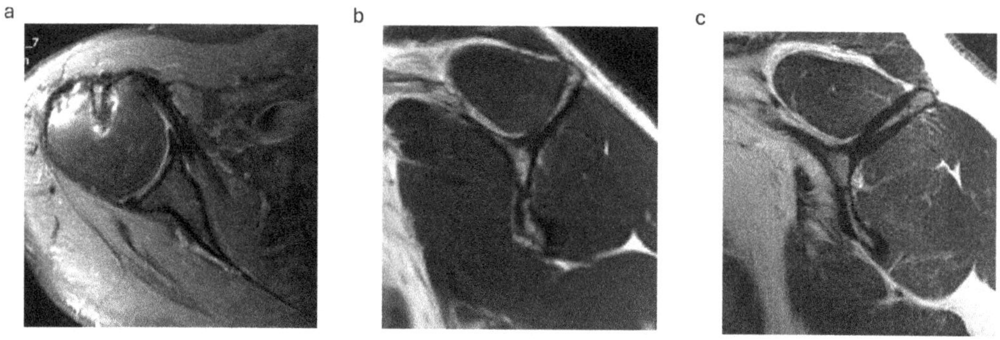

Figure 1. (**a**–**c**). Postoperative subscapularis imaging. (**a**) Intact subscapularis tendon in the axial plane (Sugaya type 1). (**b**) Subscapularis muscle with no atrophy (y-shaped plane). (**c**) Advanced subscapularis atrophy of the upper muscle portion.

2.3. Surgical Procedures

Arthroscopic repair was performed with the patient in the beach chair position. A 30°-angled scope was used through the posterior portal for confirmation of the subscapularis tear and tear grading, as well as the inspection of additional lesions, such as lesions of the long head of the biceps tendon (LHBT) or lesions of the pulley sling. The subscapularis tear size was classified according to the classification of Lafosse et al.: type II tears (complete lesion of the upper third of the tendon), type III tears (complete lesion of the upper two-thirds of the tendon) and type IV tears (complete lesion with retraction but no subluxation of the humeral head). Type I partial tears and type V tears with humeral head subluxation and combined tears of the supraspinatus or the infraspinatus were excluded from the study [5].

For tendon mobilization, footprint preparation and anchor insertion, additional anterior and anterolateral portals were established, and the subscapularis tendon edge was identified from the lateral portal (Figure 2). In the case of non-retracted tears of the subscapularis tendon, the connection to the transverse ligament was released for tear confirmation. Retracted tendons were released from scar tissue at the scapular neck, the upper tear margin and anterior scarring to the subcoracoid bursa. The mobilized tendon edge was then pulled with traction sutures to the footprint area at the lesser tuberosity.

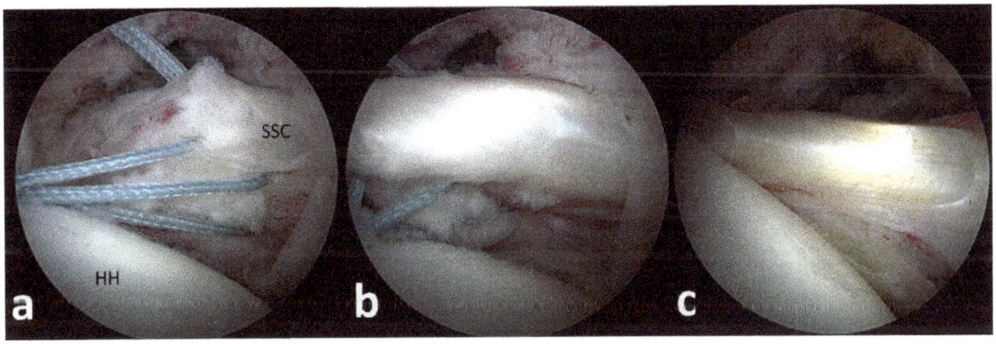

Figure 2. (**a**–**c**). Arthroscopic subscapularis repair technique. (**a**) Arthroscopic tendon identification and release of a type 3 subscapularis tear. (**b**) Arthroscopic tendon mobilization to the lesser tuberosity. (**c**) View from posterior after tendon refixation at the footprint.

The integrity and stability of the long head of the biceps tendon were inspected with a probe and graded as torn or partially torn, subluxed out of the pulley sling or completely dislocated.

Tendon refixation was performed using a single-row anchor technique with bioabsorbable suture anchors (Bio-Corkscrew® 5.5 mm; Arthrex, Naples, FL, USA), double-loaded with non-absorbable sutures (Fiberwire®; Arthrex).

Following footprint preparation, one to three anchors, depending on the size of the lesion, were placed from inferior to superior at the lesser tuberosity, and the tendons were fixed with knots after perforation with a suture passer (Figure 2, Video S1).

A dislocated or partially torn LHBT was either treated with biceps tenodesis or tenotomy according to the functional demands of the patient.

In the open repair group, a diagnostic arthroscopy was performed to evaluate the subscapularis tear configuration and concomitant lesions. Open tendon repair was performed via a deltopectoral approach with the opening of the rotator interval. The torn and retracted subscapularis tendon was released and refixed with anchors using the same surgical technique as in the arthroscopic group. Following the subscapularis repair, the LHBT was also treated with a tenodesis or tenotomy.

2.4. Rehabilitation

After surgery, the shoulder was immobilized in a shoulder sling in the neutral position for 6 weeks, and external rotation was limited to 0° for 6 weeks.

After 6 weeks, self-assisted ROM exercises and stepwise external rotation exercises were started. Patients were not permitted to perform heavy work or active exercises with the operated shoulder for 12 weeks. Active strengthening exercises with an elastic band were started after 12 weeks. After 6 months, a gradual return to their premorbid sports activity level and overhead activities of the repaired shoulder were allowed. In both repair groups, the same rehabilitation protocol was applied.

2.5. Statistical Analysis

Statistical analysis was performed using SPSS statistics software (version 26; IBM, Armonk, NY, USA), and the level of significance was set at $p < 0.05$. Data are presented as the mean, standard deviation and range. The paired t-test was used for a comparison of pre- and postoperative values. As non-parametric tests, the Wilcoxon test and the Mann–Whitney U test were used to analyze the data. For correlation analysis between samples, the Pearson and Spearman correlation coefficients were applied.

3. Results

In the ARG, 18 patients completed the final clinical follow-up at an average of 52 months (range: 48–64 months). In the ORG, 16 patients completed the final follow-up at an average of 56 months (range: 48–76 months) after surgery.

In both repair groups, most patients had a direct or indirect trauma causing the shoulder symptoms (Table 1).

In the ARG, the CMS increased from 54.1 ± 7.2 points preoperatively (range: 43–64) to 86.4 ± 6.2 points postoperatively (range: 69–99) ($p < 0.001$). In the ORG, the CMS improved from 50.4 ± 6.5 points preoperatively (range: 40–65) to 85.1 ± 6.4 points postoperatively (range: 70–98) ($p < 0.001$). There were no significant differences between the ARG and the ORG at the final follow-up ($p = 0.49$) (Table 2).

Table 2. Pre- and postoperative clinical results. CMS given in points as the mean ± standard deviation (range), and flexion and external rotation given in degrees as the mean ± standard deviation (range). Internal rotation is given as points according to the CMS, and belly-press test given as portion of positive/intermediate test results.

	Arthroscopic Repair Group (n = 18)	**Open Repair Group (n = 16)**	***p*-Value**
Constant–Murley score			
Preoperative	54 ± 7 (43–64)	50 ± 6 (40–65)	0.07
Postoperative	86 ± 6 (69–99)	85 ± 6 (70–98)	0.49
p-value	$p < 0.001$	$p < 0.001$	
Flexion			
Preoperative	128° ± 22 (63–151°)	123° ± 23 (58–155°)	0.54
Postoperative	168° ± 14 (121–180°)	164° ± 13 (125–180°)	0.31
p-value	<0.001	<0.001	
External rotation			
Preoperative	45° ± 16 (24–90°)	43° ± 18 (21–95°)	0.61
Postoperative	59° ± 9 (31–78°)	55° ± 9 (28–71°)	0.08
p-value	<0.001	<0.001	
Internal rotation			
Preoperative	5.6 ± 1.8 (2–8)	5.4 ± 1.7 (1–8)	0.63
Postoperative	7.6 ± 1.5 (4–10)	7.3 ± 1.6 (3–10)	0.59
p-value	0.001	0.001	
Belly-press test Positive/Intermediate Test result			
Preoperative	15/18 (83%)	14/16 (88%)	0.85
Postoperative	7/18 (39%)	6/16 (38%)	0.93
p-value	$p < 0.001$	$p < 0.001$	

The SST increased significantly from 5.8 ± 1.7 points preoperatively to 10.9 ± 1.4 points postoperatively ($p < 0.001$) in the ARG and from 6.1 ± 1.7 points preoperatively to 10.8 ± 1.5 points postoperatively ($p < 0.001$) in the ORG (ARG vs. ORG, $p = 0.77$).

In the postoperative course, the majority of positive or asymmetric preoperative belly-press tests and lift-off tests could be reversed by surgery or at least improved by one category, representing a significant improvement in subscapularis function in both repair groups ($p < 0.001$) (Table 2).

In the ARG, the preoperative belly-press test was negative in 17%, intermediate in 33% and positive in 50% of cases. Postoperatively, the belly-press test was negative in 61%, intermediate in 22% and positive in 17% of cases.

In the ORG, the preoperative belly-press test was negative in 13%, intermediate in 31% and positive in 56% of cases. Postoperatively, the belly-press test was negative in 62%, intermediate in 25% and positive in 13% of cases.

The belly-press test reveals a residual partial subscapularis muscle dysfunction of the operated shoulder in both repair groups, resulting in a positive or intermediate postoperative test result in 39% of the ARG and 38% of the ORG (Table 2). Postoperatively, in both repair groups, impaired subscapularis function was not necessarily correlated to a tendon retear, as there was only one tendon retear in each repair group.

Patients with a positive or asymmetric postoperative belly-press test in the ARG and ORG did not achieve lower CMSs compared to patients with a negative belly-press test ($p > 0.05$ in each group).

In the ARG, the lift-off test was negative in 56%, intermediate in 27% and positive in 17% in the postoperative course. In the ORG, there were 50% negative, 31% asymmetric and 19% positive lift-off test results. A comparison with preoperative data was not possible for the lift-off test, as the test could not be performed due to limited internal rotation in about 50% of shoulders.

In the ARG, subscapularis strength in the belly-press position improved from 2.3 (1–5) preoperatively to 4.5 (2–5) postoperatively, and strength in the lift-off position improved from 2.6 (1–5) preoperatively to 4.7 (2–5) postoperatively.

In the ORG, subscapularis strength in the belly-press position improved from 2.6 (1–5) preoperatively to 4.6 (2–5) postoperatively, and strength in the lift-off position improved from 2.5 (1–5) preoperatively to 4.8 (2–5) postoperatively.

The measurement of forward flexion and internal rotation showed a significant improvement as a result of the surgical procedure in both groups, whereas external rotation only showed only a mild improvement, mainly due to the fact that some complete type 4 tears showed excessively increased preoperative external rotation (Table 2).

The duration of the surgical procedure of 72 ± 7 min (59–91) in the ARG was not significantly longer compared to the ORG, with a duration of 68 ± 6 min (57–81) ($p = 0.15$).

An average of 2.2 suture anchors (range: 1–3) was used for subscapularis tendon refixation at the lesser tuberosity in the ARG, and in the ORG, an average of 2.4 anchors (range: 1–3) was inserted. In all cases, a complete repair with tendon refixation at the lesser tuberosity could be performed.

A lesion of the long head of the biceps tendon with subluxation or dislocation out of the bicipital groove was found in 89% (16 of 18) of the ARG. The LHBT was treated with a tenodesis in 13 cases and tenotomy in 3 cases. In the ORG, a lesion of the LHBT with subluxation or dislocation out of the bicipital groove was found in 93% (15 of 16). A biceps tenodesis was performed in 14 cases (Table 3).

Additional cointerventions were undertaken in the ARG in one case of a labral lesion with an additional arthroscopic capsulolabral repair, one coracoplasty and three subacromial decompressions. In the ORG, one humeral avulsion of glenohumeral ligaments (HAGLs) was refixed at the humeral neck, and one coracoplasty and two subacromial decompressions were performed.

As complications, there was one tendon retear of the upper portion of the subscapularis tendon in the ARG, and one retear of the upper portion of the subscapularis tendon in the ORG, both confirmed by MRI.

In one shoulder, 54 months after the subscapularis repair, a new partial bursal-sided tear of the supraspinatus was detected and treated conservatively, in addition to an intact subscapularis repair. One case of postoperative shoulder stiffness in each group in the first year after the procedure was treated conservatively and did not influence the result at the final follow-up. There were no cases of infections, anchor loosening or neurovascular injuries in both repair groups.

Postoperative MRI grading revealed one (6%) partial subscapularis retear of the cranial subscapularis tendon portion in the ARG and one (6%) partial subscapularis retear of the cranial subscapularis tendon portion in the ORG.

Subscapularis muscle atrophy grading on the sagittal MRI scans in the ARG group showed no or mild atrophy (grade 0 or 1) in 13 cases (72%) and moderate atrophy (grade 2) in 5 cases. In the ORG, no or mild atrophy was present in 11 cases (69%) and moderate atrophy in 5 cases (Figure 1b,c; Table 3).

Predominantly subscapularis muscle atrophy in both repair groups was found in the upper subscapularis muscle portion, whereas the inferior part of the subscapularis muscle was not affected significantly in these cases. Higher postoperative atrophy grades of the subscapularis muscle in both groups correlated with a higher rate of positive or intermediate belly-press tests ($r = 0.72$; $p < 0.001$). On the other hand, higher postoperative subscapularis muscle atrophy grades were not associated with significantly lower postoperative CMSs in both repair groups ($p > 0.05$).

Table 3. Surgical procedure and postoperative MRI results.

	Arthroscopic Repair Group (n = 18)	**Open Repair Group (n = 16)**	***p*-Value**
Operative time (min)	72 ± 7 (59–91)	68 ± 6 (58–81)	0.15
LHB treatment (n/%)			
Tenodesis	13/72%	14/88%	
Tenotomy	3/17%	1/6%	
Torn	2/11%	1/6%	
Subscapularis retear rate (n/%), MRI	1/6%	1/6%	
Subscapularis muscle atrophy, MRI			
No or mild atrophy	72%	75%	
Moderate or advanced atrophy	28%	25%	

Preoperative analysis of the subscapularis muscle FIG in the ARG shows an FI grade 0 and grade 1 in 89% and grade 2 in 11% of cases, with a mild progression to an FI grade 0 and grade 1 in 83% and grade 2 in 16% of cases postoperatively. In the ORG, we found a preoperative FI grade 0 and grade 1 in 81% and grade 2 in 19% of cases, with a progression to a postoperative FI grade 0 and grade 1 in 75% and grade 2 in 25% of cases.

4. Discussion

Arthroscopic repair of isolated subscapularis tendon tears achieved equivalent clinical and structural results compared to the established golden standard of open repair. The improvement in overall shoulder function, range of motion and clinical scores was slightly superior in the ARG but not significant. Subscapularis testing and structural MRI results show comparable results in the ARG and the ORG.

Given the rarity of isolated subscapularis tears and that studies with large sample sizes are also scarce, this first comparative study includes quite a large number of patients in both repair groups with a minimum follow-up of 4 years.

In the present study, arthroscopic repair achieved equivalent improvements in the Constant–Murley scores and the SST from the preoperative to the postoperative status compared to the open repair group [1,13,15,22]. Both repair techniques led to a significant regain of specific subscapularis function with a high conversion rate of positive preoperative belly-press/lift-off tests in the postoperative course [1,12,13,15,16].

Residual postoperative partial subscapularis muscle dysfunction with incomplete correction of specific subscapularis tests in about 30% of cases was observed in both repair groups [1,13,15].

As both repair groups were comparable in terms of tear size, duration from trauma to surgery and the preoperative impairment of subscapularis function (Tables 1–3), the type of surgical repair seems to not influence the residual subscapularis dysfunction. In both repair groups, impaired postoperative subscapularis test results correlated with higher atrophy grades of the subscapularis muscle detected on the sagittal MRI scans.

Both open and arthroscopic repair studies show that large tear sizes, higher degrees of tendon retraction and a longer time interval from injury to surgery, as well as advanced degrees of fatty muscle infiltration of the subscapularis, are negative prognostic outcome factors [23].

Independently of the repair technique, postoperative partial subscapularis dysfunction was not associated with significantly reduced CMS, SST or range of motion results or an increased retear rate in both repair groups [12,15,16].

Given these findings and the fact that subscapularis function is not represented very specifically in the widely used shoulder scores, evaluation of subscapularis muscle function (belly-press test and lift-off test) and correlation to the subscapularis muscle status (fatty infiltration and muscle atrophy) is mandatory to interpret the clinical and MRI results correctly, as the presence of muscle atrophy or fatty infiltration is not necessarily linked to clinical or structural failure [15,22].

In the only available retrospective comparative study, including 22 arthroscopic and 13 open repairs, Nove-Josserand et al. showed comparable CMSs (asc. group: 85 points; open group: 88 points), similar conversion rates of specific subscapularis tests with an improvement in the belly-press results in the majority of cases in both groups and a high healing rate of the subscapularis tendon on MRI scans (asc. group: 86%; open group: 92%) [12]. In their study, progression of the fatty infiltration grade of the subscapularis muscle was found in over 50% of cases in both groups and localized fatty infiltration in the upper subscapularis muscle in over 40% of cases in both groups. This increased fatty muscle infiltration was not associated with lower clinical score results or a higher tendon retear rate on MRI. Incomplete corrections of the belly-press test with a residual subscapularis dysfunction were found in over 30% of cases in both groups but were not associated with lower CMSs or a tendon retear.

Similar to these findings, we also found in this comparative study that atrophy of the subscapularis muscle was present postoperatively in about 30% of cases in both repair groups. Muscle atrophy was mainly located in the upper muscle part and was associated with an increased rate of positive/intermediate belly-press tests but not with lower CMSs or a tendon retear. The overall fatty infiltration grade of the subscapularis muscle showed slight but not significant progression on the postoperative MRI scans. The cause of this partial muscle atrophy and cases of localized fatty infiltration remains unclear and could be attributed to preoperative muscle disuse atrophy over time in combination with larger tear sizes. Other contributing factors could be an injury during the surgical mobilization procedure or increased tension status in the musculotendinous unit with loss of muscle contractility after the repair.

Gedikbas et al. and Neviaser et al. reported good clinical outcome results after the arthroscopic and open repair of isolated and combined anterosuperior tears, but the case numbers of isolated tears were too small to perform a comparison analysis between the open and arthroscopic groups [24,25].

Kamijo et al. reported superior outcome results for smaller isolated subscapularis versus larger tears following arthroscopic repair, but partial type 1 and decentered type 5 tears were also included. Larger tears showed inferior results in the ASES (American

Shoulder and Elbow Surgeon Score), a lower correction rate in subscapularis tests and a higher retear rate and fatty infiltration grade of the subscapularis detected with MRI [26]. In our study, shoulders with large complete subscapularis tears in both repair groups achieved similar clinical and tendon healing results compared to small- and medium-sized tears. This finding may be attributed to the fact that most large tears were repaired within 6 months before irreversible muscle degeneration and tendon retraction occurred [15,27].

In a retrospective multicenter study, Liu et al. presented ten-year long-term results of arthroscopic (26×) and open (9×) repair of isolated subscapularis tendon tears [28]. The study did not differentiate between the open and arthroscopic repair groups and did not include specific subscapularis tests at the final follow-up. After ten years, the study individuals reached a CMS of 75 points, which is significantly lower than our mid-term results and the average pooled results in the available meta-analysis (arthroscopic repair: avg. 84 points; open repair: avg. 82 points), but shoulder function may have declined over time. They found a comparable rate of subscapularis muscle atrophy/fatty infiltration in about 25% of cases postoperatively, which did not influence the CMS negatively and a still low retear rate of 13% after ten years, confirmed by postoperative MRI.

A hypothesis for the preserved good overall shoulder function and glenohumeral stability shown in many arthroscopic and open repair studies, with a substantial rate of persistent atrophy and fatty infiltration of the subscapularis muscle in 20–50% of cases, is that the intact lower subscapularis muscle can compensate the partial upper muscle atrophy in combination with a remaining tenodesis effect of the upper subscapularis musculotendinous unit [6,14].

In this study, we found a low retear rate of 6% in the arthroscopic and open repair groups with a single-row suture anchor repair technique. In the literature, the retear rate following open and arthroscopic repairs of isolated subscapularis tendon tears is reported as 0 to 20% [1,13,15]. These retear rates are far lower than those of isolated supraspinatus tendon tears, which is maybe attributed to the younger patient age and shorter average duration from trauma/symptom onset to surgical repair and, therefore, the better overall quality status of the subscapularis musculotendinous unit [23]. Yoon et al. reported equal clinical and structural results for an arthroscopic single-row anchor repair technique compared to a double-row repair technique for the repair of isolated subscapularis tendon tears [29].

In this study, minimally invasive arthroscopic repair with less soft tissue damage achieved slightly better score results and range of motion results compared to open repair but were not significant. Also, the duration of the arthroscopic procedure could be improved in contrast to former comparative studies, like the UKUFF trial that reported a significantly longer operative time for arthroscopic repair [30]. In this study, the duration of the arthroscopic procedure was not significantly longer than that of the open repair procedure. On the other hand, the costs of arthroscopic rotator cuff repair are reported to be higher than those of comparable open repair procedures due to specific arthroscopic instruments, fixation devices and single-use instruments [30]. In this study, we can report a significant improvement in the shoulder outcome scores (CMS and SST) in both groups. The arthroscopic repair group achieved equal improvements looking at the MCID (minimal clinically important difference) and the SCB (substantial clinical benefit) of the clinical scores from the preoperative to the postoperative status [31].

This study has several limitations. First, it was a comparative, prospective study with no randomized patient assignment, and the MRI assessment was not blinded. The statistical power of the study was limited by the relatively small number of subjects. As strengths, we performed a uniform tendon fixation technique in both groups, and the outcome assessment was performed by assessors who were not members of the surgical team. A potential advantage of arthroscopic subscapularis repair is that concomitant intraarticular injuries, like capsulolabral lesions, can be addressed directly, and less soft tissue damage and scarring leads to faster regain of a range of motion and lower rates of shoulder stiffness in the early postoperative course.

5. Conclusions

In summary, we found in this first comparative study that arthroscopic repair achieved equivalent clinical mid-term results compared to open repair. Also, tendon healing and the muscle status of the subscapularis, as detected by MRI, showed comparable results following both repair techniques. Arthroscopic subscapularis repair can also be considered a surgical standard for the rare and complex entity of isolated subscapularis tears.

Supplementary Materials: The following supporting information can be downloaded at: https://www.mdpi.com/article/10.3390/jcm13216589/s1, Video S1: Arthroscopic subscapularis repair.

Author Contributions: Conceptualization, C.B., F.G. and S.P.; methodology, C.B., F.G., S.P. and S.E.; investigation, C.B., F.G., S.P., J.D. and L.H.; writing—original draft preparation, C.B. and S.P.; writing—review and editing, C.B., F.G., S.P., J.D. and S.E.; visualization, C.B., S.P. and S.E. All authors have read and agreed to the published version of the manuscript.

Funding: This research received no external funding.

Institutional Review Board Statement: This study was conducted according to the guidelines of the Declaration of Helsinki and approved by the Ethics Committee Ulm University protocol reference number 192/14 on 28 July 2014.

Informed Consent Statement: Informed consent was obtained from all subjects involved in this study.

Data Availability Statement: All data are contained within the article.

Conflicts of Interest: Author Stefan Eichhorn was employed by the company Tüv Süd. The remaining authors declare that the research was conducted in the absence of any commercial or financial relationships that could be construed as a potential conflict of interest.

References

1. Mall, N.A.; Chahal, J.; Heard, W.M.; Bach, B.R., Jr.; Bush-Joseph, C.A.; Romeo, A.A.; Verma, N.N. Outcomes of arthroscopic and open surgical repair of isolated subscapularis tendon tears. *Arthroscopy* **2012**, *28*, 1306–1314. [CrossRef] [PubMed]
2. Bedi, A.; Bishop, J.; Keener, J.; Lansdown, D.A.; Levy, O.; MacDonald, P.; Maffulli, N.; Oh, J.H.; Sabesan, V.J.; Sanchez-Sotelo, J.; et al. Rotator cuff tears. *Nat. Rev. Dis. Primers* **2024**, *10*, 8. [CrossRef]
3. Lee, S.H.; Nam, D.J.; Kim, S.J.; Kim, J.W. Comparison of Clinical and Structural Outcomes by Subscapularis Tendon Status in Massive Rotator Cuff Tear. *Am. J. Sports Med.* **2017**, *45*, 2555–2562. [CrossRef]
4. Bartl, C.; Scheibel, M.; Magosch, P.; Lichtenberg, S.; Habermeyer, P. Open repair of isolated traumatic subscapularis tendon tears. *Am. J. Sports Med.* **2011**, *39*, 490–496. [CrossRef]
5. Lafosse, L.; Jost, B.; Reiland, Y.; Audebert, S.; Toussaint, B.; Gobezie, R. Structural integrity and clinical outcomes after arthroscopic repair of isolated subscapularis tears. *J. Bone Jt. Surg. Am.* **2007**, *89*, 1184–1193. [CrossRef]
6. Rathi, S.; Taylor, N.F.; Green, R.A. The upper and lower segments of subscapularis muscle have different roles in glenohumeral joint functioning. *J. Biomech.* **2017**, *63*, 92–97. [CrossRef]
7. Labriola, J.E.; Lee, T.Q.; Debski, R.E.; McMahon, P.J. Stability and instability of the glenohumeral joint: The role of shoulder muscles. *J. Shoulder Elb. Surg.* **2005**, *14* (Suppl. S1), 32S–38S. [CrossRef]
8. Gerber, C.; Hersche, O.; Farron, A. Isolated rupture of the subscapularis tendon. *J. Bone Jt. Surg. Am.* **1996**, *78*, 1015–1023. [CrossRef] [PubMed]
9. Edwards, T.B.; Walch, G.; Sirveaux, F.; Mole, D.; Nove-Josserand, L.; Boulahia, A.; Neyton, L.; Szabo, I.; Lindgren, B. Repair of tears of the subscapularis. *J. Bone Jt. Surg. Am.* **2005**, *87*, 725–730. [CrossRef]
10. Heuberer, P.R.; Smolen, D.; Pauzenberger, L.; Plachel, F.; Salem, S.; Laky, B.; Kriegleder, B.; Anderl, W. Longitudinal Long-term Magnetic Resonance Imaging and Clinical Follow-up After Single-Row Arthroscopic Rotator Cuff Repair: Clinical Superiority of Structural Tendon Integrity. *Am. J. Sports Med.* **2017**, *45*, 1283–1288. [CrossRef]
11. MacDermid, J.C.; Bryant, D.; Holtby, R.; Razmjou, H.; Faber, K.; Balyk, R.; Boorman, R.; Sheps, D.; McCormack, R.; Athwal, G. Arthroscopic Versus Mini-open Rotator Cuff Repair: A Randomized Trial and Meta-analysis. *Am. J. Sports Med.* **2021**, *49*, 3184–3195. [CrossRef] [PubMed]
12. Nové-Josserand, L.; Hardy, M.-B.; Ogassawara, R.L.N.; Carrillon, Y.; Godenèche, A. Clinical and structural results of arthroscopic repair of isolated subscapularis tear. *J. Bone Jt. Surg. Am.* **2012**, *94*, e125. [CrossRef] [PubMed]
13. Saltzman, B.M.; Collins, M.J.; Leroux, T.; Arns, T.A.; Griffin, J.W.; Romeo, A.A.; Verma, N.N.; Forsythe, B. Arthroscopic repair of isolated subscapularis tears: A systematic review of technique-specific outcomes. *Arthroscopy* **2017**, *33*, 849–860. [CrossRef]
14. Burkhart, S.S.; Tehrany, A.M. Arthroscopic subscapularis tendon repair: Technique and preliminary results. *Arthroscopy* **2002**, *18*, 454–463. [CrossRef]

15. Rinaldi, V.G.; La Verde, M.; Coliva, F.; Cammisa, E.; Lullini, G.; Caravelli, S.; Mosca, M.; Zaffagnini, S.; Muccioli, G.M.M. Arthroscopic approach does not yield better results than open surgery after subscapularis repair: A systematic review. *Knee Surg. Sports Traumatol. Arthrosc.* **2023**, *31*, 2688–2699. [CrossRef]
16. Bartl, C.; Salzmann, G.M.; Seppel, G.; Eichhorn, S.; Holzapfel, K.; Wörtler, K.; Imhoff, A.B. Subscapularis function and structural integrity after arthroscopic repair of isolated subscapularis tears. *Am. J. Sports Med.* **2011**, *39*, 1255–1262. [CrossRef]
17. Constant, C.R.; Murley, A. A method of functional assessment of the shoulder. *Clin. Orthop.* **1987**, *214*, 160–164. [CrossRef]
18. Lädermann, A.; Collin, P.; Zbinden, O.; Meynard, T.; Saffarini, M.; Chiu, J.C. Diagnostic Accuracy of Clinical Tests for Subscapularis Tears: A Systematic Review and Meta-analysis. *Orthop. J. Sports Med.* **2021**, *27*, 23259671211042011. [CrossRef]
19. Fuchs, B.; Weishaupt, D.; Zanetti, M.; Hodler, J.; Gerber, C. Fatty degeneration of the muscles of the rotator cuff: Assessment by computed tomography versus magnetic resonance imaging. *J. Shoulder Elb. Surg.* **1999**, *8*, 599–605. [CrossRef]
20. Samim, M.; Beltran, L. The Postoperative Rotator Cuff. *Magn. Reson. Imaging Clin. N. Am.* **2020**, *28*, 181–194. [CrossRef]
21. Sugaya, H.; Maeda, K.; Matsuki, K.; Moriishi, J. Functional and structural outcome after arthroscopic full-thickness rotator cuff repair: Single-row versus dual-row fixation. *Arthroscopy* **2005**, *21*, 1307–1316. [CrossRef] [PubMed]
22. Monroe, E.J.; Flores, S.E.; Chambers, C.C.; Zhang, A.L.; Feeley, B.T.; Lansdown, D.A.; Ma, C.B. Patient-reported outcomes after isolated and combined arthroscopic subscapularis tendon repairs. *Arthroscopy* **2019**, *35*, 1779–1784. [CrossRef] [PubMed]
23. Rhee, Y.G.; Lee, Y.S.; Park, Y.B.; Kim, J.Y.; Han, K.J.; Yoo, J.C. The outcomes and affecting factors after arthroscopic isolated subscapularis tendon repair. *J. Shoulder Elb. Surg.* **2017**, *26*, 2143–2151. [CrossRef] [PubMed]
24. Gedikbas, M.; Ozturk, T.; Erpala, F.; Zengin, E.C. Comparison of Open Versus Arthroscopic Repair for Subscapularis Tendon Tears With or Without Concomitant Supraspinatus Tendon Tears. *Orthop. J. Sports Med.* **2022**, *10*, 23259671221120662. [CrossRef]
25. Neviaser, A.S.; Charen, D.A.; Cotter, J.M.; Harrison, A.K.; Cagle, P.J.; Flatow, E.L. Retrospective review of open and arthroscopic repair of anterosuperior rotator cuff tears with subscapularis involvement: A single surgeon's experience. *J. Shoulder Elb. Surg.* **2020**, *29*, 893–897. [CrossRef]
26. Kamijo, H.; Sugaya, H.; Takahashi, N.; Matsuki, K.; Tokai, M.; Ueda, Y.; Hoshika, S. Arthroscopic Repair of Isolated Subscapularis Tears Show Clinical and Structural Outcome Better for Small Tears Than Larger Tears. *Arthrosc. Sports Med. Rehabil.* **2022**, *28*, e1133–e1139. [CrossRef] [PubMed]
27. Lanz, U.; Fullick, R.; Bongiorno, V.; Saintmard, B.; Campens, C.; Lafosse, L. Arthroscopic repair of large subscapularis tendon tears: 2- to 4-year clinical and radiographic outcomes. *Arthroscopy* **2013**, *29*, 1471–1478. [CrossRef]
28. Liu, Y.; Lafosse, L.; Opsomer, G.; Villain, B.; Kempf, J.F.; Collin, P. Ten-year clinical and magnetic resonance imaging evaluation after repair of isolated subscapularis tears. *JSES Int.* **2020**, *6*, 913–918. [CrossRef]
29. Yoon, J.S.; Kim, S.J.; Choi, Y.R.; Kim, S.H.; Chun, Y.M. Arthroscopic Repair of the Isolated Subscapularis Full-Thickness Tear: Single- Versus Double-Row Suture-Bridge Technique. *Am. J. Sports Med.* **2019**, *47*, 1427–1433. [CrossRef]
30. Mohammed, K.D.; Lloyd, R.F.W.; Nagaraj, C.; Krishnan, J. The Relevance of Open Rotator Cuff Repair in 2021. *Indian J. Orthop.* **2021**, *55*, 433–442. [CrossRef]
31. Cvetanovich, G.L.; Gowd, A.K.; Liu, J.N.; Nwachukwu, B.U.; Cabarcas, B.C.; Cole, B.J.; Forsythe, B.; Romeo, A.A.; Verma, N.N. Establishing clinically significant outcome after arthroscopic rotator cuff repair. *J. Shoulder Elb. Surg.* **2019**, *28*, 939–948. [CrossRef] [PubMed]

MDPI AG
Grosspeteranlage 5
4052 Basel
Switzerland
Tel.: +41 61 683 77 34

Journal of Clinical Medicine Editorial Office
E-mail: jcm@mdpi.com
www.mdpi.com/journal/jcm

www.ingramcontent.com/pod-product-compliance
Lightning Source LLC
Chambersburg PA
CBHW062106220926
51850CB00010B/2913
* 9 7 8 3 7 2 5 8 6 6 2 2 9 *